Eric —

you are also
an inspiration of
Health to me.

Stay Healthy +
Stay Successful!

M000169697

PRAISE FOR

BRAINLESS HEALTH

"John Patton brings a new, important voice to health communications. John's work with the National Association of Chronic Disease Directors and the Centers for Disease Control and Prevention (CDC) offers common-sense best practices for living a better life fueled by health. John uses personal stories of humor, spirituality and health science to bring his 'health hacks' to the forefront in a well laid out and layered book of practical actions.

"*Brainless Health* and the multitude of resources found within will provide the reader with a guide to finding 'your best you.' I knew after reading it the four or five areas I needed to improve. He writes in a fun-loving way of storytelling that will leave the reader wanting for volume II."

—JOHN ROBITSCHER, CEO, National Association of Chronic Disease Directors

"John Patton delivers with *Brainless Health.* Life's journey may have derailed some of us from making all the best health choices, but John Patton's passion, deep insights and personable writing style lets us know it's not our fault and it's never too late to make healthy choices."

—DAVID IRISH, Director CBSHealth, Business Development

"This book helps us all lead healthy lives easily, without overthinking. This is not about weight loss and muscle building but just feeling healthier and better. Packed with tips on food, sex, exercise, loneliness, and even money, *Brainless Health* is written not by a medical expert but someone who spends every working day creating simple, plain-language messages for our nation."

—**STEPHEN MURPHY**, Director WebMD, Public Health Solutions

"I couldn't be happier to recommend this book. John Patton offers the reader some down-to-earth wisdom focused on living a healthier lifestyle based in common sense and actions that can fit into our lives. I encourage you to read this and think!"

—**DR. DAVID HOFFMAN**, Associate Dean for Academic Initiatives, Maria College

Brainless Health:
Simple Health Habits for Smart People

by John William Patton

© Copyright 2020 John William Patton

ISBN 978-1-64663-024-0

All rights reserved. No part of this publication may be reproduced, stored in a retrieval system, or transmitted in any form or by any means—electronic, mechanical, photocopy, recording, or any other—except for brief quotations in printed reviews, without the prior written permission of the author.

Published by

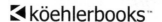 köehlerbooks™

210 60th Street
Virginia Beach, VA 23451
800-435-4811
www.koehlerbooks.com

JOHN WILLIAM PATTON

BRAINLESS HEALTH

SIMPLE HEALTH HABITS FOR SMART PEOPLE

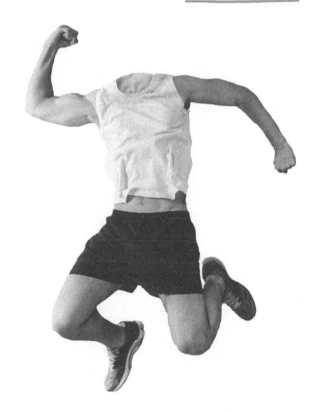

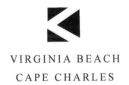

VIRGINIA BEACH
CAPE CHARLES

TABLE OF CONTENTS

PREFACE

GOOD HEALTH IS NOT that hard. It really isn't.

Unless you had a childhood disease, you were probably pretty good at being healthy when you were a kid. You probably went to bed early and got up early. You probably ran around at recess and had a physical education or gym class. You ate what was cooked for you and it likely included a few green items. You had orange juice and milk and soda only on occasion. You rode a bike or ran around outside after school. You got the common cold, but in general, you were probably healthy.

We can't go back to those days, but we can admit that staying healthy wasn't exactly rocket science. You didn't count your carbs or any other macro or micronutrients. You didn't worry about your gut health and you couldn't spell *turmeric*. Those things aren't bad; they are just hard to integrate into a busy life. *People are not dumb, they are busy.* Very busy. We are so busy that remembering to log our meals, charge our step tracker, weigh our food or even remember to carry our water bottle can become a challenge. That's especially true if you are up late working (or binging on Netflix), dealing with a colossal commute, or dropping off family members at day care, after care or elder care. Perhaps your increasing need for faster and faster food has caused you to be on a first-name basis with the kid at the drive-thru. Or maybe you have sitting disease. You are chained to your desk chair all day, then you sit in your car to drive home, only to sit at the dinner table and finally sit in your favorite recliner in front of the TV.

It's no one's fault that the modern age snuck up and took our health hostage. But it is our responsibility to take it back.

This book will help you do that. But it is not only for you. Don't be selfish. Be sure to share it. Give it to everyone you know. I'm serious. Photocopy it if you must. It's for your mother and your father. It is for your employer and your neighbor. It's for your kids and your friends and your kids' friends. That's because smart people everywhere are doing stupid things that sabotage their health, wealth and happiness without even knowing it. Education, wealth or the number of followers you have on social media do not guarantee health. In fact, they often run counter to a life of health and fulfillment. Smart people with plenty of money and lots of social media stimulation often find themselves on the couch, having their dinner delivered while texting videos to their friends who are doing the very same thing.

This book is called *Brainless* because there are truly brainless things you can do, and *absolutely must do*, to keep yourself out of wheelchairs and free from feeding tubes, oxygen tanks and nurses lifting you onto the toilet.

Virtually every book on health and wellness is way too technical or hard to follow for more than a week. Their principles are too demanding, too time consuming or just too darn boring. While volcanic sea salt is truly amazing, who has time to learn about it, measure it, mix it, track it or, frankly, remember to buy it?

Add to our crazy, busy lives the dizzying debates around the basic foods that we eat. The constant confusion causes *health paralysis*. Let me illustrate.

Below is a list that I generated in five minutes off the top of my head. It focuses *only on food*, but we could make a similar list for just about any area of health and wellness. I call it the *Confusion*

Illusion. That's because, while it is indeed confusing, it is only an illusion that all healthy choices require scientific debates. This book is all about things that are *not* debatable because they have been proven to work. Period! But go ahead and chuckle at this familiar list of confusing topics. Don't worry about any of them until you have mastered *everything* in this book. That's job one.

Caffeine versus decaf
Saturated fats versus unsaturated fats
Splenda versus Aspartame
High fat versus low fat
Added sugar versus natural sugar
Whole grain versus multi-grain
Low carb versus no carb
Whole eggs versus egg whites
Egg whites versus eggbeaters
Butter versus margarine
Plant protein versus animal protein
Omega-6 versus omega-3
B6 versus B12
Healthy fats versus bad fats
Dairy versus non-dairy
Vegetarian versus vegan
Goat cheese versus cow cheese
Diet soda versus regular soda
Red wine versus white wine
Smoothies versus cold-pressed juices
Energy drinks versus energy shots
Complex carbs versus simple carbs
Good nuts versus bad nuts
Gluten versus gluten-free
Organic versus sustainable
Farm raised versus wild caught
Cage free versus free range

Whew! Today, our emerging health culture is more robust than ever—and more apathetic than ever. We can become numb to what is healthy and what is not. Today's superfood is tomorrow's cancer-causing agent. What increases my risk for disease suddenly becomes my savior. The endless questions can often cause us to throw in the towel and just order another beer.

Meanwhile, easy stuff that you don't have to think about promises a foolproof path to health and happiness. That's my point; that's what I'm here to share. No debates allowed. These are timeless truths that will deliver better returns than Warren Buffet could ever do in the stock market.

While running our busy lives, we simply don't have time to become doctors, dieticians or personal trainers in order to get healthier.

As titillating as fad diets and infomercials are, we just don't have time to educate ourselves about trace minerals, probiotics, or even green tea. The good news is that you don't need to know the benefits of beet juice or beef stock. That's because you already know a ton about what to do to stay healthy and get happy. You just need to do it. You need to *do* what you already know to do.

By the way, let's be clear. Without *physical* health, you can kiss goodbye riches and relationships. Without health, you are going to be seriously challenged when it comes to succeeding in life. How are you going to get promoted at work when you are a sneezing sack of sickness, constantly taking time off to go to the doctor? How are you going to be there for your grandkids when you need oxygen just to climb the bleacher steps to watch their game? And I hate to say it, but I'm sure it's hard to kiss goodnight with a CPAP machine strapped to your face. Think about it. This is real life. These are real issues and they are only the tip of the iceberg.

So, before we get too far down the line, let me be clear. I have serious sympathy for the sick and broken in society. That's exactly why I'm writing this book. I look at the landscape of society's bodily bedraggled and I weep. Many of them had *nothing* to do with their condition or got the news too late to change their health. That is a devastating reality. What's far worse, however, are the people who *can* affect their future and who are doing nothing. They are dying by 1,000 paper cuts. They are letting every excess calorie and every extra minute on the couch kill them. Period. The message of this book is for those who still *can* change the course of their life and avoid needless suffering in their child's basement apartment or nursing home.

On top of the can of whoop-ass that I hope to deliver, I will give you a path to develop healthy habits that will work in the background of your life, automatically, while you pick up the kids, attend the meeting, clean the house, buy the groceries, wash the car, walk the dog and go out with your friends.

This book is a gold mine. It provides no-brainer health hacks that are so logical and easy to follow that you will dramatically reduce your risk of experiencing a life of suffering and misery while dramatically increasing your health and happiness. I guarantee it.

So, get ready to get healthy, *without even thinking.*

CHAPTER ONE

GET OFF
THE COUCH

IF YOU'VE NEVER HEARD of me, relax. You are not here because of me, but because of what I must share with you.

If you must know why I'm the perfect person to bring you extraordinary insights into what you *should* already know, I'm a professional health communicator. I get paid to communicate health for a living, and that qualifies me as an expert in the field. Please note, however, that I am not a doctor. I am not a nutritionist. I am not a dietician or a personal trainer. I am the guy who tells you to drop your cigarette, wash your hands, put down your fork and step away from the plate, take your dog for a walk, guzzle some water, wear a helmet, and start acting like you care about your health and the people you love.

I am the guy who works with smart people in the government who research what makes you healthy and what keeps you healthy. My colleagues are geniuses with doctorates in medicine, public health and related fields. They often speak in ways that most people can't understand *or simply don't care to understand.* These science geniuses have big vocabularies to go with their big hearts and big brains. Their language can be confusing or discouraging. They use words like *physical activity* instead of just saying *exercise* and *physical inactivity* instead of saying *sitting on your butt.*

The very fact that I don't have a PhD and I don't do longitudinal research studies or write medical articles makes me the perfect person to talk to you in ways that avoid medical jargon and confusing acronyms and abbreviations. I cut to the chase of how to get healthy. But that's not why I decided to write this book.

INSANE BEHAVIOR

Over my last ten years of working in public health, I have had to pussyfoot around health communication in order to be inclusive, non-judgmental and politically correct, yet all the while watching people of all socio-economic, ethnic and sexual orientation fall off the deadly cliff of disease and disability instead of protecting themselves with completely brainless healthy behaviors. I literally watch thousands of people not washing their hands, not applying sunscreen, only taking the stairs if the elevator is broken, and shoveling tons of food down their throat long after they are pleasantly full.

The only explanation I can come up with for this insane behavior, despite constant health messaging, is that *they simply don't know the risk of their actions.* Of course, they know that they should eat healthy and exercise, but they feel fine. After all, it's Friday and they feel like a beer or an ice cream or a *frappasugarccino.* Heck, it's been a long week, so let's go to the movies and order the refillable popcorn bucket with the refillable soda.

Maybe you're stressed out or anxious. Maybe you just deserve a break today. Or maybe you are young and feel invincible. Maybe you are getting older and you have survived this long, so there's no need to change what seems to be working.

Whatever the reason, people everywhere are oblivious to the raging waterfall that is right around the bend in the river. It doesn't matter your age or stage in life. Sadly, they don't know that a few simple actions could prevent a lifetime of pain and suffering. That's what I'm talking about—*suffering, not death*. I'm talking about horrible decades of nastiness that makes people beg for death.

Whenever I hear people say, "Well, you've gotta die of something" as they light up another cigarette, I cringe. Or what about "A little dirt isn't going to kill you." They are simply clueless; a little bit of the *wrong dirt* could in fact kill you or just introduce you to a friendly tapeworm that will make you vomit and convulse and never go out to a restaurant again. *Hello?*

These days, I eat healthy and exercise. But I didn't always. About ten years ago, I was far from healthy. I ate a donut every day and I drank alcohol every night. At one point I kept a bottle of tequila front and center on my desk. I was a beast. I would treat myself to an ice cream cone most nights *before* dinner. Thanks to McDonald's pervasive jingle, I believed that I really did deserve a break today and *every* day.

Then, I woke up and decided that I was "sick and tired of being sick and tired," as author Bill Phillips famously said. I decided to change my lifestyle so that I would feel better when I went to bed and feel better when I got out of bed. Plus, I wanted to look better, improve my confidence at the beach and start to walk the talk at my job.

Unfortunately, I quickly discovered that the internet and infomercials did little to bolster my health comprehension. It was difficult figuring out what the doctors and experts wanted me to do to achieve healthy results. I had no idea what to do, where to do it or how to do it.

And so, I turned to the health and fitness influencers, the beautiful people on social media who make a living selling supplements and teeth whiteners. But the more I tried to find out which amino acids I needed in my diet and how to perfectly balance my macronutrients, I discovered that the experts agreed on very little. They were touting the newest preworkout or the latest branch chain amino acid. Since no one agreed, I didn't know whose advice to follow. I didn't have the education or the time to get educated.

That's when I decided to focus on the things that pretty much everyone *does agree on* and are rarely debated. They are the actions and diets that every mother teaches her kid.

DEBATABLE HEALTH

This book cuts through what I call *debatable health* to help you focus on the brainless things that no one debates. They have already been proven for decades, if not centuries, to positively impact your health.

If you are tempted to think that most people already know everything in this book, just ask yourself why so many people waddle when they walk. Ask yourself why US obesity rates are at a record high. Ask yourself why heart disease is the number one killer, yet 80 percent of strokes are preventable according to the Stroke Awareness Foundation. Ask yourself why we spend $10 billion on antacids annually. *Hello?* Ten billion for *one* condition closely related to diet. Is anyone paying attention? Has anyone got an answer?

Maybe you personally don't waddle, but do you loosen your belt after dinner? Do you polish off the bag of chips, the box of cookies or the bottle of wine on a semi-regular basis? Do you sleep but don't feel rested? Do you know you should exercise but you want to lose weight *first* so you look better in your spandex at the gym?

Back in the day, no one was obese because they either couldn't afford food or they worked so hard it burned right off their body. Today the American Medical Association has declared obesity a disease and it has been labeled an epidemic, something that is often preventable.

You will learn things that you either didn't know before or never thought about in an accessible way. It's likely that you are not following most of these brainless behaviors and that you have no idea how powerfully they can decrease your risk for chronic diseases and an overall life of disfiguring pain and disability. Likewise, you have no idea how much health and happiness, vigor and vitality await if you adopt these simple practices.

But first, I want to be crystal clear about how I define the word *health*. Health isn't just the absence of disease or sickness. Even the healthiest people get sick. They get food poisoning, the flu, strep throat . . . etc. The difference is that healthy people get better *faster.* They rebound faster. They get off the medications faster. They feel better sooner and for longer amounts of time between sicknesses because their immune system is high functioning. They feed themselves with health and fuel their muscles with strength.

When debilitating diseases like cancer come calling, doctors will tell you that people who are in shape and otherwise healthy bounces back from chemo faster and battle the cancer cells with greater efficiency and success. It just makes sense, but it's something we often don't consider when we are feeling good. We think we will always feel the way we feel when we are healthy. *Wrong!* Illness has your number. It is coming for us. Our job is to be prepared and beat it away.

Health also applies to our mental, emotional, financial and relational life. Heck, you can be a cover model and miserably alone and forgotten. Maybe no one calls you because you are a relational moron. Maybe you never learned to have healthy relationships and value people. Maybe you are paranoid or critical and judgmental. Maybe you are anxious and fearful and that is impacting your sleep. Maybe you are alone because you never thought you needed anyone. Maybe you never learned to save money and now you are in horrible financial health, which is wreaking havoc on your physical body, relationships, work . . . etc. There are tons of reasons that you may be sick due to horrendous health in your head or heart. Good news. This book is here to help.

HEALTHY FUTURE

First, you have already watched enough Netflix. Way too much. I have too. It's time to turn the channel to your health and your future. Your health is the single greatest determiner of whether you will see your kids graduate, see them get married, see another elementary school soccer match, piano recital or karate kick fest. Your health will likely determine whether you get that job or promotion, whether you will be able to travel the world now (or after you retire) and whether you'll have to outfit your home with tubes, monitors and a bed on wheels.

If you want to live a long, happy life so that you can go to the ball game, keep your teeth in your head (without glue) and breathe without wheezing, then you have to make decisions about your *future* health—today.

I'm not talking about positive thinking or hoping for the best. I'm talking about deciding, determining and declaring that you will begin to make healthy choices in your life every day, starting now.

Throughout this book I emphasize "tend to your health or your health will need tending to." Here's a perfect analogy:

We all want our cars to run well and not break down. But how many of us take the time to learn about our car's engine, watch YouTube videos about mufflers or radiators or, heaven forbid, read the manual that came with our vehicle? But we can all remember to change the oil every 3,000 miles without much thought. That's because Jiffy Lube marketed that message to us thirty years ago and it made sense. So now we just do it and our cars thank us by running a lot better and longer. Most of us don't know *why* an oil change helps our car run better and we don't really care—we just do it. Sure, our cars still break down, and so will our bodies, but not nearly as often (or as badly) as they would if we ignored simple maintenance. Hospital stays, just like visits to the auto mechanic, can be avoided.

It's a simple fact that a lot of people are going to the hospital and dying every day—needlessly. They are living with chronic conditions and taking buckets of pills that cripple their ability to remember things, get out of bed, go to the bathroom, walk, talk or even fall asleep.

The news media and politicians love to quote our nation's astronomical healthcare costs, but rarely do people connect the dots between dollars and disease. High costs mean *high suffering*, and if you don't know someone with a debilitating, devastating disease, then just go spend a day in a hospital waiting room. Just show up and look around. No one will kick you out. Just watch the wheezing and the coughing. Count the wheelchairs and see the swollen limbs and puffy eyes. Most of all, try to find a smiling patient. Tubes and needles and bed sores make for sadness and misery.

We all know that it sucks to have the flu. Try having the flu every day of your life for twenty years. That's what chronic means. Daily suffering is what defines *chronic* illness, *chronic* disease and *chronic* pain.

Western culture has a way of hiding the sick and suffering in the corners of communities, in the hospitals, nursing homes, rehabilitation facilities and basement apartments. Sometimes we see a little old lady in the grocery store in a motorized cart and it doesn't bother us much. But rarely do we see her try and get into her car, or into her home, or out of bed. We don't see her struggle to get to the bathroom. We don't see the plateful of pills she takes or the diarrhea that they cause her.

Moreover, we don't see the person blinded by Type 2 diabetes or a housebound husband suffering from a stroke or someone with an amputated limb. Nope. Those folks typically don't show up on our way to school or work or the mall.

None of those horrors will ever happen to you, correct? I get it, you are busy, happy and successful. You feel good today. You probably don't stress about your health because you have better things to do than spend hours trying to figure out how to stay out of the hospital and off the meds. You are focused on getting through the day or having a good night. You work hard and deserve to take a break.

The good news is that you don't have to work hard or spend very much time to massively impact your health if you take advantage of the simple ideas in this book. You just need to change your own oil every 3,000 miles and you can keep on truckin'.

That's because a lot of diseases in America are 100 percent preventable. Sure, cancer gets a lot of attention and it is a ravaging, non-discriminating disease, but even cancer has its own set of prevention practices. The National Foundation for Cancer Research reports a reduction in breast cancer simply by exercising regularly. Ask anyone who has had their breast removed whether they would trade regular trips to the gym for regular chemo treatments. Of course, you can do everything right and still take an arrow to your heart (or breast), but reducing the risk is what this book is all about and what everyone's life should include.

Healthy living isn't about living like a monk or carrying your salad to work in plastic containers. Nor will it make you into a bikini model or prepare you to climb Mt. Everest (although it could do both). Rather, it will start you on a path to integrate simple, real-life changes into your daily life that will foster real improvement. It will help you embrace the ancient Greek definition of health as *the place between self-indulgence and self-neglect.* In other words, you can still be the *life of the party* and *remember the party* in the morning.

A WORD ABOUT WEIGHT

In case you were skimming any of my golden words, I want to remind you that this book does not relate *health to weight.* I don't know what your weight is, but I know that if you live in the Western world, you probably think a whole lot about your weight. You may even obsess over it. (Eighty percent of Americans do, according to *The Huffington Post.*) Moreover, you have likely been brainwashed to believe that the words *health* and *weight* are synonyms, which is incorrect.

The medical community invented the confusing term *healthy weight*. I'm not here to debate the docs; I just want you to know that there are millions of skinny sick people and plenty of heavy, healthy people according to the terribly flawed Body Mass Index (BMI) weight scale. So, when it comes to food, this book is about brainless ways to improve the quality and quantity of the food you eat—not how much you weigh. Let's focus on the *quality* of your weight and not on the *quantity* of your weight.

Note: Your weight can be important, but living a healthy lifestyle is job one, and typically weight loss (if needed) will be a natural byproduct.

HEALTHY HABITS

Fundamentally, the hardest part of forming any habit is remembering to do it, and typically, the key to remembering something is to make it easy to remember. Make it simple, logical and memorable. We tend to remember things that make sense, and if it rhymes, all the better.

If we must engage our brains too much, we usually fail. That's why I try to steer clear of that in this book. Fear not; If you want to look up the facts and figures, go for it. There are tons of statistics and studies to back up every assertion in this book; but that's not my focus. This book is designed to create knee-jerk responses, not contemplative cognition or debate.

This book doesn't require understanding complex medical opinions or statistics or trends. I won't ask you to measure your food, log your carbs or count your drops of sweat. I will tell you to *just do it.* Follow my instructions. Act. Do. Implement brainless, blind adherence to time-tested truths and, *violà*, you will be healthier and happier.

To help you achieve these goals I'm going to be part coach and part drill sergeant, and 100 percent your best friend. If you do what I say, you will win the battle for your life. That's right; it's a battle every day.

Every time you see a festival food truck offering deep-fried Twinkies®, remind yourself that it is a frontal attack that's gunning for your arteries. When you see online ads for extramarital affairs, remember that they are coming for your marriage and your family. When you see *no interest for thirty-six months,* remember that the company is in business to grow its bank account, not yours. Get it? This is a war and the enemy is serious. It will ravage your health and happiness.

One last note on the war analogy. We all have seen movies and documentaries of how soldiers are broken down and disciplined during their basic training so that they will robotically follow orders in the heat of battle. They snap to attention at the sound of a whistle and fly into action at the sound of a bullet. That is because in battle *you don't have time to think.* You must react to save your life. There's no time for debate or second guessing.

The goal of this book is to train you to build habits that are so ingrained in your skull that you just do them. When you open a menu at a restaurant or you flush the toilet or your alarm goes off in the morning, you just act. You know what to do and you do it.

To prove just how insidiously subtle the war on our health can be, I recently landed in Las Vegas for a health conference. I jumped into a cab at the airport and told the driver to take me to the hotel. Within minutes he asked me if I wanted to swing by the cannabis dispensary to pick up some marijuana. Imagine that! The driver even said he could get me to the front of the line. I'm in the back seat asking myself where the hidden camera is. I'm asking myself, *Why in the world is this guy trying to get me to buy weed?* Gone are the days of sketchy dealers on the corner pushing dope. Now it's the average cab driver!

Fortunately, I'm not a pothead, and drugs are not on my bucket list, but there are a ton of people who visit Vegas every day who will be easy targets for a dope-pushing cab driver. I'm not a prude. I know the stats and I know the risks and I know that neither are worth it.

The impact of drugs on your body are real. Get your highs elsewhere. Don't screw with your health.

If you want to do weed, thrilling. I'm not judging anyone for anything in this book. My goal is for you to understand that it's not healthy to fill your lungs with *any kind of smoke*. Period. Moreover, it isn't healthy to fill the air around you with smoke, especially if you have kids, pets, roommates or family that live with you. You can debate me all day long, but I'm not taking the bait. That's not my purpose here. Rather, it is to make sure you know that life is a legitimate battle, and if you can remember easy, logical, lifesaving tips, then you will increase your chances of staying alive, chewing with your original teeth and preventing the use of adult diapers for as long as possible.

WHY TRUST THIS GUY?

As I mentioned earlier, you are probably wondering who I am and why you should follow my lead. Let me share that I have spent the last decade working in public health, and believe me, I know about the health of the public. It's not pretty. I have also worked more than twenty years in the field of communications, media and marketing, and for the last decade, I've been communicating about health for the National Association of Chronic Disease Directors and working with the Centers for Disease Control and Prevention (CDC).

I've spent thousands of hours inside the CDC's hallowed halls hearing about the state of our collective health and helping to inform the public. Today, I serve as the executive director of the ProVention Health Foundation, which works to prevent disease and disability. My work has focused on the biggest chronic diseases, from heart disease to diabetes to cancer, trying to communicate life-and-death messages to the general public. It's painfully hard because of the politics of government, red tape, clearance and the need to never offend anyone—even if it could save a life. In this book, I am unfettered from those bonds, so believe me, I will speak freely.

At the end of the day, I wrote this book because I am done with sitting on the sidelines. I am ready to empower people with no-brainer action items that will make a mountain of difference in their lives.

I look forward to your feedback. I know that changing behavior can be daunting and breaking old habits can seem impossible. Fortunately, it's a lot easier when someone shoots straight. I hope you view me as someone who truly cares about helping you live healthier, happier and longer. Let me know what works and what doesn't, and maybe together we can help even more people improve their life by improving their *health*, brainlessly.

CHAPTER TWO

FINDING YOUR WAY

FIRST THINGS FIRST. We must establish your *why*. That's what author Simon Sinek says, and he's a pretty smart guy. So, let's go with that. Why get healthy? Why change your behavior? Why read this book? Why become a health evangelist? Why integrate health into every single area of your life?

Only you can answer those questions. And let me suggest that your *whys* should be ambitious but sustainable. If you just want to lose a few pounds, fit into a wedding dress or look better at your high school reunion, then there are tons of books, pills, machines and surgeries to help you. Conversely, if you want to feel better every single day, improve your relationships, fatten your wallet, excel at work, increase your confidence, sleep better and think clearer, then you have to articulate your *why*.

When temptation comes knocking (and it will), remember why you are changing your life. Why you are *choosing* new choices that you never chose in the past. Why you care about things you didn't care about before. *Why you are building brainless health habits that will effortlessly guide the rest of your natural life.*

Maybe it's because you want to be around for your daughter's wedding and the grandkids that may come afterward. Maybe you want to travel without a walker when you retire and visit places that don't accommodate wheelchairs. Maybe it is so that you can avoid erectile dysfunction and not strain the golden years of your marriage. Just decide and write it down on paper and on your heart.

MY WHY

The ocean might just be the greatest symbol of health and relaxation in the world for me. The year was 2014 and I sat on the beach feeling the breeze skim off my bald head and the sun bronzing my sun-screened face. I could hear the waves crashing and lapping against sand.

That morning, I began with a walk along the beach, followed by a quick workout in the hotel gym that overlooked the ocean. It was a refreshing workout, but not a straining, grueling workout that makes one dizzy and want to puke. It was a short and simple regimen that sent oxygen into my lungs and blood early in the morning to fire up my metabolism and clear my head. I followed it up with a double espresso, a mimosa and some pancakes. (Hey, I was on vacation.)

My point in sharing this scene is that this picture has become my personal picture of health. I mixed some early morning discipline with some tasty indulgence.

In order to enjoy a vacation like this, I need to be able to walk *to* the beach and walk *along* the beach without excruciating pain or someone helping me out of my wheelchair. I need to be comfortable taking off my shirt in public and able to enjoy my espresso without causing heart palpitations. I need to enjoy pancakes without worrying about my high cholesterol or creating an elevated glucose reading. Finally, I need to enjoy the warmth of the sun without the fear of skin cancer.

That's *my* personal picture of health. Yours might be the ability to garden in your yard and then drink fresh lemonade with real sugar on a sun-drenched porch without an insulin pump or a bunch of pain killers to ease the soreness from kneeling in the dirt for hours. Maybe you want to throw the football with your son or nephew on a cool fall day and enjoy the smell of fresh cut grass without having an asthma attack. Maybe your picture of health is simply being able to sleep through the night and wake up refreshed without using sleeping pills and enduring their side effects. *Now picture the opposite and wince.*

Whatever your picture of health is, think about it. Take a minute to paint the picture and then embrace it.

Decide you are going to do everything in your power to make healthy, smart decisions. Simply define health for yourself and then fixate on it. Don't compare yourself to anyone else. Rather, compare feeling bad to feeling good. Then decide that it is time that you started feeling good, refreshed, rested, confident, energetic, attractive, empowered to take life by the horns. Or for starters, simply decide that you are ready to feel comfortable after a big meal or after you climb a few stairs.

Remember, I'm not prescribing a fitness regimen or a special weight loss plan. I'm not Tony Robbins or Brian Tracy or any other self-help genius. This is a book about brainless health, not medical health or perfect health or beautiful health, but smart, easy, simple health that prevents disease and disability. I'm not a doctor or a witch doctor. I am a busy person trying to grab a vacation in the middle of raising a family, going to work and paying the bills. I'm an average Joe trying to enjoy eating out and going to the movies while staying out of the hospital and feeling as good as possible after the meal and the movie are over.

I'm also a guy who has done it. I'm not bragging, I'm testifying. It's possible and it's worth it.

VISUALIZE YOUR HEALTH

So, start by imagining your own picture of health. Write it down or print out a picture of it and stick it *in* your refrigerator (not on the front but *inside the fridge*). Yep. Put it on a sticky note or laminate it, and stick it somewhere *inside* your refrigerator because, firstly, food will have a huge impact on whether you reach your goal, and secondly you will likely see it every day if it is inside your fridge. The goal is to visualize your health and then be reminded of it regularly. I know people who find a picture of what health means to them. Maybe it is a person or a place. It might be a grandkid or a beach house or a foreign city or a delicious donut that you want to be able to enjoy without guilt or gout. Seriously, we don't even consider the little joys in life, like favorite foods, that can suddenly become off limits if you get diagnosed with a nasty disease.

Get moving! Job one, find a sticky note or picture. Job two, stick it inside your fridge.

UNFORTUNATE REALITY

Sadly, I meet many people who honestly don't care about their health. They hate the hassle of having to take antacids or go to the doctor, but it is a small inconvenience in comparison to their love of cigarettes, Big Macs and television.

I really can't wrap my head around it, and it is hard for me to believe it, but I see it all of the time. You do too. Maybe you can relate. Maybe your wife or husband begs you to quit smoking, to change your unhealthy habits, but you just don't. You just won't. You just don't want to. You just don't care. Enough!

The only way I can begin to understand that mentality is that the person in question must simply not know what is coming. They don't think about going to the pharmacy every week or traversing the grocery store trolling an oxygen tank behind them. They haven't even been to a dialysis center, let alone had the treatment. They don't consider not being able to drive, or living on one floor because they can't go up the stairs by themselves. They have never had to sort pills on the kitchen counter and spend half their day putting them into plastic containers with the days of the week on them just so they don't overdose by mistake.

Of course, most people think it will never happen to them. My son said as much; everyone thinks they are immune. But they are dead wrong, and the tiniest bit of education will prove it. It's funny that people play the Power Ball lottery believing that they will win when the odds are 1 in 175 million. Conversely, the chances that you already have prediabetes are one in three. Believe the math if you don't believe me.

I was on a film shoot for a prediabetes TV campaign in LA and I talked to one of the team who had conducted the focus groups prior to the shoot. She said that all that they wanted a particular man in a focus group to simply say that he would *consider* going to the doctor to find out if he had prediabetes. The man refused and wouldn't even utter the words. He wouldn't make a promise he knew he wouldn't keep. He said that he already knew he probably had prediabetes. He knew he was overweight. He knew what the doctor would say; therefore, why go in for a screening? Why waste his time and his doctor's time? I'm sure that a lot of people can relate.

Going to the doctor could turn up something you don't want to know about. That's a common reaction and a common fear. When it comes to health, people believe that ignorance *is* bliss, that no news is good news. Unfortunately, nothing could be further from the truth. The real, terrifying thing is *not knowing* what is lurking below the surface. The thing to be afraid of is *not* finding out if something is wrong until it is too late, and you wake up with a catheter and colostomy bag.

Let's be crystal clear. No one with stage-four cancer will tell you that they are glad they discovered it late. No one, ever.

I recently spent an hour talking to a used-car dealer who told me story after story about how his doctor has tried to help him. His wife, a nurse, begged him to stop smoking. He had diabetes and angioplasty surgery to unclog three out of his four blocked arteries.

The salesman told me that he went to a diabetes self-management class. He said he learned a little bit about how much sodium is in the foods that he continues to eat. But at the end of the day, he said that he didn't want to give up fast food. He told me that there was a Whole Foods within walking distance of his office, but that it would take too long to get his food and pay for it. Instead, he explained that he can order ahead at the burger joint and have his assistant pick it up for him, so he wouldn't have to leave his desk.

In the middle of his soliloquy, while bragging about how efficient he was at getting his fatty food choices *delivered* right to his desk, he completely missed the fact that his little plan was eliminating even the smallest amount of exercise. His sedentary lifestyle was wildly increasing his risk for heart attack and stroke. *Double death—* nutritionless food plus zero exercise.

The salesman acknowledged that his doctors had to give him pills to deal with his current health issues, but that the drugs lead to horrible side effects such as numbing his facial features, excruciating neck pain and even a burning penis. (I'm not kidding. It was an incredibly awkward conversation to have with a stranger on a used car lot).

He even told me how the smoke from his cigarettes had ruined his designer reading glasses by creating a yellow tint to them. But *even that* did not deter him. (I can't make this stuff up.)

I told him that he would likely drop dead in the very near future or that he would soon be climbing aboard the slow train of suffering, complete with ventilators, dialysis and loss of vision. (Think about that. It sucks to be confined to your bed as you are dying, but just imagine not even being able to watch TV because your diabetes took your eyesight.) That's what we are talking about here, and it happens every single day.

At the end of the conversation the salesman said that he already knew that all he needed to do was change his lifestyle. He knew the exact path to health. He knew that lifestyle alone could possibly lead him off medications and prevent him from going blind, having his toes amputated or having a stroke. He just wasn't interested. He wasn't ready. End of story. I get it. I really do. Stages of change are real, and he simply wasn't willing to make the change at that time.

DON'T DELAY

The really bad news is that none of us will be in a better position to change *later* than we are right now. It's just a brainless fact. Every single day, we get older and closer to death. Every day we get stiffer and more immune deficient. We will have more nicotine in our blood, more cholesterol in our arteries, weaker knees and less energy to start the changes needed. Every day we get slower. Every day that we delay making the necessary changes, *the harder those changes will be.*

While that salesman may seem to be an extreme example, there is a little bit of him in many of us, including myself. *We know exactly what to do, we just don't want to do it.*

So, what exactly will we do in the meantime? What will make us do the work? Get with the program? Take responsibility? Just freaking do it? Answer that question. Take a second to identify your barriers. Your problems. Your excuses.

A friend of mine, who is always reading the latest book on flavonoids, tannins, neuroplasticity, and every other health breakthrough, recently answered that exact question by telling me that each person must have their own *ah-ha* moment.

He went on to tell me about a man he met who was a couch potato until one day, while watching the Olympics on television, a marathon runner inspired him to change his life. The very next day, the man began to run. He couldn't even run around his neighborhood once.

In a relatively short period of time, he started running marathons and today he is training for an ultramarathon (100-mile road race).

That's an amazing story and I've heard plenty of them. So have you. Likely you have envied them. One's ability to change is admirable. A woman wakes up one day and decides she wants to stay alive to walk down the aisle of her granddaughter's wedding. Another person decides they want to hike the Grand Canyon. Another person loses a family member and decides to end the cycle of disease in their own family.

I love those stories, *but I am not really interested in them*. That's because I'm not interested in waiting around for people to have their own special, *ah-ha* moment. I'm not interested in people waiting for a family member to drop dead before they decide to get off the couch. I'm not interested in one more excuse that puts off a life-or-death decision for one more day.

MOBILIZING

My personal vision is a nation of people collectively saying, *"Enough is enough."* Neighbors asking each other if they want to start walking in the morning together. Coworkers asking the boss if they can get a water cooler for the office or asking if the company will help subsidize gym memberships instead of their cellphone bills. I am interested in people asking their doctors if there is a lifestyle-change program instead of a pill that they can take. I am interested in family members clearing out the junk food from their pantry and deciding to stock up on healthy alternatives. I am interested in whole communities that vote for bike lanes and walking paths and parks. I'm looking for a neighborhood, office, community and world like that.

Thank goodness that entire nations have decided that racial segregation is wrong and that a college education is brilliant and that protecting the environment makes sense. What I want is a seismic shift in culture that shuns fast food and embraces hiking. I want the next generation to treat their bodies like the amazing creations that they are, naturally and respectfully, without even thinking about it. I am interested in a world where people *always* choose health.

It's not hard once people discover that they feel better (mentally, physically and emotionally) after deploying health-conscious behaviors instead of pain numbing, destructive behaviors (like smoking, binge drinking and hyper-caloric eating). It can happen if people give it a try. That is my vision. That is my real *why*.

CHAPTER THREE

HEALTH IS THE NEW BLACK

DESPITE NEON COLORS, FALL florals and spring hues, in the fashion industry black is always the bomb. It is slimming and goes with everything. So, everything wants to be the *new* black. It is the gold standard in clothing.

Well, good news; *health* is the new black. Health makes you look slim and makes you *feel* slim. Health goes with everything from evening wear to sportswear. Health is fashionable cocktail conversation and good in the bedroom. Health is about confidence and sleeping well. It is about clearer and tighter skin. Health helps your bank account and your relationships. It is way better than black—*by far.*

For years, the fashion model was the desired body type, those skinny types that nobody could become without mental or physical disorders. Then came the fitness model, which was a step in the right direction. It was about strength and being limber. It was about low body fat and firm muscles. It gave birth to the CrossFit craze. Gyms opened on every corner, and then they got their own CrossFit games. It was sexy and successful, but still was rather unattainable for the masses. It was hard to sustain while raising a family or traveling for work. Finally, *health* became the term *du jour*, and its arrival was a bright spot in history. *Health* was more about the inside instead of the outside. It was harder to compare, but easier to measure. You knew if you were *being healthy* even if no one could see it. You knew the choices you were making. You knew what you were eating and how you were exercising. You knew your cholesterol, blood pressure and glucose numbers, and for the first time you felt empowered to control them. Being in the driver's seat of your health meant that you influenced the quality of your life and the quantity of your years. Add to that, Madison Avenue and Wall Street are finally on our side. Big business discovered that *health* is big business.

We are living in a great new world of health. Bottled water, once the joke of the party, is now the star of the party. Fiji and Vox vie for star power like champagne or Scotch. And how about gluten-free everything? From beer to cookies to protein bars, you can avoid gluten whenever you want (if that's your thing). And now there is exercise for everyone. There is yoga and hot yoga and even goat yoga. There is Zumba and body aerobics, Pilates and barre, and a zillion different kinds of spin classes. There are rowing gyms and even surfboard gyms. There are climbing walls and climbing gyms. There are hiking and walking and running clubs. You can find fitness equipment on the beach and in parks and along wooded trails. There is even an outdoor free-weights gym under an overpass in NYC.

There are paths for bikes, roller blades and skateboards. There is an unlimited product market of health equipment from jogging strollers to rubber-coated dumbbells. There are juice bars and cold-pressed vegetable drinks. There are literally dozens of coconut waters, not to mention milks made from coconut, almond, soy, rice, cashew, and hemp.

GNC and The Vitamin Shoppe now face major competition from regular grocery stores. Entire aisles are being devoted to protein powders, squeeze gels, power drinks and nutrition bars. Even my favorite pizza parlor now lists meat toppings under the heading *proteins.*

It's vogue to eat sushi, go to a salad joint, order up a quinoa bowl or order your burger with a lettuce bun. In other words, health has finally climbed society's ultimate market rung—*respect.* People respect healthy people who make healthy choices. That alone is reason to embrace *health.* Here is a fun example.

I knew a man who raised his kids based on the health principles that he practiced. One of his famous behaviors involved parking in the farthest spot from the front door of the grocery store or mall. That way he always found a spot and he got exercise walking to the entrance. Of course, his children complained bitterly, but he was teaching them through his own life choices. Later in life, he had a dream that he died and his children parked the hearse in the farthest space from the church just so they could honor his legacy. I love that story because I deeply believe that the choices we make today can affect the next generation.

More important is that we can affect the next generation *by staying alive to love them* and spend as much time with them as possible. Who wants to hear their grandfather say that he can't go to the baseball game or dance recital because walking is too hard for him? Plus, when you are in pain, you get grumpy. That's why a lot of older adults are mischaracterized as angry. They are just in pain. Moving around hurts. Swallowing hurts. They don't sleep well, and they get tired very quickly. That's if they aren't proactive and stay in shape long before they become old. I always aim to be the kind of grandparent that is "out-hiking" his grandkids.

If we can practice great heath then the next generation will respect us, learn from us, and want to emulate us. We will show them that health is always the new black and it is always in style.

CHAPTER FOUR

THE ELEVATOR IS BROKEN

THE OTHER DAY, I went to work, and the elevator was broken. It was like a car wreck on the highway. I've never heard so much grousing and complaining and rubbernecking around the closed steel doors. You'd think people were being asked to walk across hot coals. Most didn't even know where the stairs were. I on the other hand was upset because my typically vacant access to my office was jammed with wheezing whiners.

I normally have every stairwell to myself at any time of the day. I often walk up to the tenth floor when I feel like exercising in the middle of the day, usually before lunch or during that three o'clock lull. Sometimes I take my conference calls while walking the stairs. Why not? It's so simple, and it's *brainless*. Why sit when I could be exercising my heart and strengthening my muscles? Yes, I have an exercise ball in my office and I sometimes do sit-ups while I'm on conference calls too, but taking a walk is a whole lot easier and I don't get as winded.

But for some reason we are conditioned not to take the stairs. Some of my female colleagues avoid the steps because of their high heels. Others, however, embrace it as a chance to strengthen their calves and enhance the shapeliness of their legs. I don't wear heels, so I really can't comment except to say that millions of New Yorkers dress in heels, but they also walk to work in sneakers. Anyone can do that. Even my male colleagues bring sneakers to work and change into them for an afternoon walk. Many people live in walk-up apartments, without elevators, and so traversing stairs is a regular part of their life. They throw on their joggers in the morning with their business suit and then change their shoes once they hit the boardroom. Sure, it takes effort. Sure, it takes planning, but it's pretty brainless and the health payoff is massive.

Speaking of New Yorkers, the next time you are in a New York subway, count the escalators in the subway. That's right, there are very few. People don't complain and they sure haven't stopped taking the trains. They just do it. Up and down every day, multiple times a day, and as a result you see a lot fewer obese people in New York City, despite the amazing restaurants and food carts on every single corner.

Each time I go to any airport, I stop to photograph the completely empty staircases that flank the escalators jammed with people. I'm not talking about escalators jammed with suitcase-carrying people, but rather people who are headed to *claim* their suitcases, and those with no suitcases at all. They have just finished sitting for hours on a plane, consuming peanuts and cookies and sodas. Yet, once deboarded, they refuse to exert any more energy than is absolutely required.

If you must take the escalator, try walking on the moving stairs. You'll get to your destination faster while exercising. Try it at the mall, the hotel and at the convention center. And for goodness sake, walk down it if you can't walk up it!

The moving sidewalks are the greatest commentary on our culture of obesity. Except for the elderly, these contraptions scream laziness. I always walk next to them and race the people on them. Without breaking a sweat, I beat them every time. I'm not bragging and I'm not talking about getting to point A faster than my fellow travelers. I'm talking about seizing a golden opportunity to move through an airport while burning a couple of the calories I just ingested on the airplane.

I can imagine 1,000 years from now, archeologists will uncover a moving sidewalk and scratch their head wondering what on earth humans were trying to move with these contraptions. Only when they excavate millions of obese people will it dawn on them that they were transporting themselves.

Once you start looking for stairs, you will find them. Parking decks typically have great signage for the elevators and typically the stairs are next to them. In shopping malls, it can be harder to find them, but they're usually anchored on the ends of the mall, and some feature beautiful, sweeping designs. I play a game of asking retail clerks that come to their job at the mall every day where the stairs are. Very few have any idea. In hotels, taking the stairs is downright efficient, especially if you are headed down. If I were king, I'd make it mandatory to take the stairs *down*. Down is brainless. Down is easy. Down doesn't even make you sweat, but at least you are moving your muscles and joints in ways that you wouldn't otherwise.

Whenever I go to a hotel, I ask for a low floor so that I can use the stairs to go up. It removes the stress of waiting for the hotel elevator, which typically gets crowded and then seems to stop on every single floor.

Always check the door in a hotel stairwell before closing it behind you. In some buildings, there are fire doors and security systems that automatically lock the stairwell doors (go figure) to keep people from having access. Sadly, I speak from experience. I locked myself and my children in the stairwell of a hotel, which was solid concrete, thwarting even the strongest cellphone signal. We had to walk to the bottom of the hotel to find the emergency exit onto the street. (Let's just say my kids learned a life lesson.) All the health in the world isn't worth getting stuck in a building's stairwell.

Another tip is to go to the bathroom on another floor of your office building. This is so crazy simple. Just hike up or down a few floors every time you want to use the restroom. Then keep increasing the floors if you have the time (and if you won't wet your pants in the meantime.) As an added benefit, you won't stink up the bathroom just when one of your colleagues walks in. Sometimes I walk all the way from our second-floor office to the tenth floor of my building because the bathrooms there are much nicer.

My fitness club is on the top floor of an outdoor mall. I used to drive up to the top of the parking deck and walk straight into the gym. Then I realized that I could exit the parking deck a heck of a lot faster if I parked on the first floor and walked up the three flights to the gym. It acts as a pre-workout warmup and keeps me from getting stuck in a long line of cars trying to exit the deck.

Now don't get me wrong; taking the stairs is not always a picnic. For some reason, no matter how many miles I jog, even two flights of stairs can leave me winded. I presume it is because stair climbing engages different muscles than running, which holds an altogether additional health benefit.

My sister is a physical therapist and she works with the elderly on balance and strength issues. One of her favorite exercises to prescribe for patients is to walk up four stairs and back down again every day, three or four times a day. *Not four flights* of stairs, just four stairs. This simple activity addresses muscular, skeletal and cognitive skills. You engage your brain for balance when using the stairs. If walking the stairs is too much for someone, my sister will have them perch on one stair with half of their foot hanging off, in order to stretch their calf muscle while practicing their balance.

My friend's mother went from playing tennis every day to sitting in a wheelchair in just six weeks once she moved into a home with an elevator and stopped having to use the stairs in her home. That punctuates the utterly mind-blowing power of stairs.

Think of stair*wells* as stairs *to* wellness. Stairs will make you well *if* you take them.

CHAPTER FIVE

FOUNTAIN OF YOUTH

I REALLY CAN'T ADDRESS this next brainless activity any better than Dr. Mike Evans in his YouTube video titled *23 ½ Hours*.

It's worth watching at least *twice*, then share it with everyone you know. Dr. Evans is a medical doctor, and like any physician, he has zillions of drugs and therapies at his fingertips that reduce risks for heart disease, stroke, diabetes, arthritis and even cancer. But before prescribing drugs, he usually tells his patients *to walk* thirty minutes a day regardless of their health condition. That leaves people with *23 ½* hours to watch TV, sleep, eat, go to work, go to the bathroom, pick up the kids, surf the internet, and post on social media.

It's completely brainless. Just dedicate yourself to walking your dog for thirty minutes. Listen to an audio book while you walk. Call your aging parents, or kids in college. Call an old friend. Find a walking partner. Power walk around the grocery store or around the mall. (If you didn't know it, a lot of malls open early, before the stores open, just for walkers.) Walk to the store, to the bus, to a neighbor's house or to a friend's office on another floor in your building. Park in a parking lot away from your office and walk to your office. Many offices charge a lot for parking, and if you can find a free lot (or cheaper lot), just walk from there. You'll be helping your heart and your wallet.

Walking can be a great form of meditation or prayer or simply resting your mind from the barrage of emails and phone calls and texts. I often use walking or running as a time of peace and reflection. Sometimes I leave my phone at home when I walk or go to the gym just so I can process life without interruption. That simple behavior of putting down your phone for thirty minutes a day can be a health benefit. (Be sure to tell someone where you are going if you don't take your phone.)

When it comes to walking, I am personally indebted to the fitness trackers of the world like Fitbit® and Polar® and Garmin® and Apple® for pushing step-trackers into a socially acceptable (and even enviable) space by making them both functional and fashionable. I often read articles that challenge the accuracy of step-tracking devices and I am always amazed.

No one seemed to care that the old-fashioned two-dollar plastic pedometers of yesteryear weren't precise, but now that they are super high-tech, easy to use, sync with your phone and track 100 other biometrics, everyone is suddenly a critic. For goodness sakes, if they only make you more *aware* of your approximate level of physical activity (and inactivity), we've won! I'm amazed at how often I stare down at my Fitbit® only to discover that I've barely walked 2,000 steps all day. I really don't care if I've walked 2,100 steps or 1,900 steps. The point is that I haven't been moving. Similarly, whether I hit 9,800 or 10,000 steps a day (CDC's recommendation), I don't care because I know that I'm killing it. I'm moving. I'm active. I'm helping my heart. I'm helping my body. Period.

Business guru Peter Drucker said, "If you can't measure it, you can't improve it." Smart man.

Now, of course, many of these companies have gotten pretty darn good at being pretty darn precise with their technology, and that is all the better, especially when it comes to tracking heart rate and sleep, two critical health variables in addition to physical movement. It is also great that they have improved their accuracy because every company in America seems to be doing some kind of company step-challenge or competition of one kind or another. Wellness teams are handing out gift cards and blenders and movie tickets and cash prizes to the people or teams that walk the most. There are apps and websites and dashboards to track the steps of each member of the team. There's nothing like a little healthy competition to get healthy. My colleagues and I often remind each other that it doesn't matter how someone gets healthy, just that they do.

Of course, like anything, moderation is the key. One day I was on business in San Francisco and decided to take a walking tour of the city with my boss. We went farther than expected, and by the time we returned for dinner we had walked 39,000 steps. After bidding him goodnight, I walked another five laps around Union Square just to reach 40,000 steps (approximately 20 miles) to set my own new personal best.

TRUE STORY

Similarly, my brother-in-law got a Fitbit for Christmas one year and threw down the gauntlet and challenged my wife and me to a couple's step-challenge. The goal was to see which team could walk more in the course of one month. Since we were all using Fitbits®, we could know how each other was doing, minute by minute. Therefore, before the first week was up, my brother-in-law and I were out for blood. He would get his wife out of bed at night to go play an hour of ping pong just to increase their combined step count. Similarly, my wife and I were running every day together. On many occasions, I would hit the gym after work, and stay on the treadmill until the gym closed. I would listen to Spanish language podcasts, audio books and even watch entire football games all while running or walking on the treadmill. Needless to say, our competition got out of hand fast, and by the third week, my brother-in-law had developed a bone spur from hours of running up and down the stairs in his home. Finally, he threw in the towel and I couldn't have been happier. I got a great steak dinner out of the competition, but I'm happy to buy my own steak from now on.

Nevertheless, I'm still a big fan of step-tracking devices. Today, steps are a kind of social currency. I meet people and they see that I am wearing a tracker and they ask about my number of steps today. Therefore, do not treat a wearable device like jewelry. Walk the walk. These devices scream, *"I care about my health."* They can also be an incredible career-building tool. What business owner or boss wouldn't want to see employees investing in devices to improve their health?

If you are scratching your head about how to get in some extra steps while living in this driveway-to-parking lot world, I've got some tips. Try parking at Macy's at the mall if you are going to Bloomingdales. Try shopping at a different grocery store so you will have to walk your legs off trying to find where bread and pickles are located. Try parking on the highest floor of the parking deck and taking the stairs. Park in your own garage at home and then walk back down the driveway to get your mail. While you are there, look through your mail while you walk up and down your street. Still challenged? Schedule your next phone call while you walk. Talk and walk. Tell your colleague in advance that you are planning to walk during your next conference call and won't be in front of your computer. Ask if that is OK. You can still tap out any critical notes on your phone if needed. *We must get creative, and we have to start to change the culture around us.*

My CEO used to go for a walk in the middle of the day. He would send out an email to everyone in our office thirty minutes before he left and invite anyone to join him. It was a simple, easy, brainless move to give people the inspiration (and permission) to leave their desks and exercise.

Of course, we all know that people in Europe walk more than Americans because their towns and cities are more compact, and they have been doing it forever. It is a learned behavior that kids just accept. Plus, gas is typically more expensive, and sidewalks abound.

Recently, I met one of my new neighbors. She and her husband arrived straight off the ski slopes of Switzerland. After a few minutes chatting with the wife, we said goodbye and I walked to my car. I had no sooner fired up my engine and peeled out of the neighborhood than I spotted her walking to the grocery store with a small backpack on her shoulder. I was stunned. Nobody left our neighborhood on foot. It's practically a crime. On top of that, she was headed toward the grocery store. Even for me, walking to our grocery store would never cross my mind. (Among other reasons, I doubt I could successfully hoof it back with a bottle of Tide, a gallon of milk and a bag of dogfood over my shoulder.) But for her, it was natural. It was a way of life. It was a beautiful day and she was getting some exercise while getting some groceries. Brilliant, and brainless!

I know a man who, at age ninety, had brain surgery from a head trauma. I asked him if he was able to still take walks, and he indignantly said, "Of course I do. I only walk half a mile, but I do it every single day!" He also said that he did thirty sit-ups and ten push-ups each morning. He was the picture of health, conversant and independent, doing his own home repairs and taking cross country vacations with his grandchildren. That's what I want for myself at ninety.

Doctors said that his physical fitness was the key factor in his speedy recovery from brain surgery. He will be the first to tell you that *walking* is the fountain of youth.

CHAPTER SIX

GOALS YOU CAN MEASURE

BEFORE BECOMING HEALTH CONSCIOUS, I was a rat. What I mean is that I ate like a rat. I ate just about everything and anything in the house, or in the hotel lobby, or at grocery store food sample stations. I'd pick up cookies at the rental car registration desk or finish off the last piece of birthday cake in the office breakroom. I'd tilt my head back and empty the remaining potato chip crumbs. I always told myself it was *just one* Girl Scout cookie or *just one* spoonful of ice cream, or *just one* (more) beer. I would literally sniff out leftovers in the refrigerator between meals and finish off the fries from my kids' plates at restaurants. Yes, I was a rat, and perhaps you are too.

Then I became a different kind of rat when I joined a gym. Fear not, I didn't become *that kind of gym rat*. I didn't start spending hours every day at the gym, making friends in the gym or flexing in front of the mirror, but I did *join* a gym and I started to go every Monday, Wednesday and Friday. I still often only show up for thirty minutes or even just fifteen, but I have committed to go regularly. Just *go* to the gym. I didn't say *work out*. I promised myself that I would show up. Whether I stay there and work out or turn around and go home, I committed to showing up. That may sound crazy, but it works like a charm.

Of course, what happens 99.9 percent of the time is that once I get to the gym, I end up working out. I know that there is zero chance of exercising if I stay at home, so by going to the gym I at least have the *possibility* of exercising.

When I first started, I couldn't run a mile. Now I can run six miles easily and typically run three miles a day.

I used to have a long commute to work, so I'd leave around 5 a.m. and drive forty-five minutes to the gym, work out, shower and then go to the office. Other times, I'd be so exhausted that I would drive to the gym, park, climb into the backseat and go back to bed. But at least I made it to the gym. I treated it exactly the way I treat brushing my teeth. It's what I do when I get out of bed.

If you want to do it on the way home from work, that's fine. If you want to work out at lunch, that's fine. Just make it automatic. Completely brainless. DO NOT play it by ear and go to the gym if you *don't* have lunch plans or *if* you get off early. It will get cancelled. If you do it at lunch, put it on your calendar and refuse calls or meetings during that time. If you do it after work, leave your office at 4 or 4:30. Make it a requirement.

One survey, by CreditDonkey® (that's really their name), stated that 80 percent of people who join a gym in January stop going by May. It is also reported that 4 percent of people who join gyms in January stop going *in* January. I get it. I really do. I was like that.

So, that's why I now just tell myself to wake up and get to the front door of the gym. Five years later I'm playing the same game with myself. I wish I could tell you that I jump out of bed with a smile. I rarely *ever* want to go. When I am running late it is even worse. But I do it just to force myself to feel the pressure and inconvenience and pain of being rushed so that I will remember it the next time I am tempted to hit the snooze button.

Going in the mornings is best. There are typically fewer people who go in the morning, which means I don't have to wait to use equipment. Also, there are fewer things that are going to get in the way of me going. Plus, the mornings seem to be full of slightly more serious fitness people. Someone once told me that the people in the morning are there for results and the people in the evening are there to socialize. Of course, that is an unfair generalization, but there is typically more socializing going on after work at the gym, and it is usually twice as crowded.

Statistically, almost half of all people go to the gym with a friend. I love that statistic and I greatly encourage you to find a friend who will go with you because they will keep you accountable. Accountability is the number one way to stick to any goal or commitment. Period. If you don't have a friend to work out with, then tell a friend *about* your commitment. My buddy Andy goes to a jujitsu gym and wrestles with other grown men at 6 a.m. He holds me accountable. I will often snap a picture of the sunrise outside my gym and text it to him to let him know that I made it to my gym. We are invested in each other's life, not our egos.

Note: I talk about this later in the book, but it's worth repeating: *You are going to look and feel like the people you hang around.* This is so powerful. Find friends who value what you value. Find people who inspire you and link up with them. Go to lunch with them. Go to 5K races with them. Go shopping with them. Whether you are out to dinner or on a cruise or at the gym together, they will rub off on you in positive ways.

If you can go with a friend to the gym, they can help you navigate how to use various pieces of equipment without the awkward feeling that everyone has experienced trying to figure out where your head goes and where your feet fit. Going to the gym with a friend is also efficient. Whether you are walking on the treadmill together or making sure the bench press doesn't crush each other's sternum, it is a great way to catch up with old friends or build a new friendship. I know many people from my neighborhood who are workout-friends. One day they simply noticed the other person walking in the morning or mentioned that they belonged to the gym, and before you know it, they are exercising together. Knowing that your friend will be waiting for you at the gym or at the entrance of your neighborhood will get you out of bed on a cold morning. Social interactions, such as the ones that friendships provide, also improve one's overall mental and emotional health.

Economically speaking, in the past, gyms were only for middle-to-upper income earners and were typically located in the suburbs, but today there are gyms on every corner that charge small fees with no long-term financial contract or commitment. In fact, if you don't have $10 a month to invest at a place like Planet Fitness® for the sake of your health, then you have a bigger problem than this book can address. I encourage you to spend *more* than $10 a month on your body because no other investment will pay dividends like investing in your health.

You need to view your gym, yoga studio, YMCA membership, or tennis shoes as serious financial investments. If you ignore that investment, you should feel like a complete moron. After all, Apple Music costs $10 a month. As much as I love my music, my health is at least 10,000 times more important to me. In fact, if you are paying $10 or $20 a month *for anything* and not investing in your health, don't tell anyone.

OK, buckle up. Here comes the heavy sales pitch.

I'm a big fan of walking and running outdoors as I said earlier. But everyone within five miles of a gym should join and here is why.

Unlike the benefits of walking and taking the stairs, a gym allows you to work out your *total body*. As we age we lose muscle mass and bone density. This leads to horrifying diseases such as osteoporosis, which creates brittle, weak bones. Half of adults sixty-five and older will experience a serious fall. Falling leads to broken bones that either don't heal correctly or lead to other illnesses while recuperating in the hospital.

I used to think that the *50 percent fall* statistic meant that old people need to pick up their feet and try not trip on the carpet, but the reality is that many people fall because their bones are so weak that they break while they are still standing and that causes them to fall. *Hello!* If you are an older adult, you know that the very last thing you need to add to your life is a wheelchair, cast or crutches.

While there is no shortage of machines to give you a good aerobic workout at a gym, from elliptical machines to rowers to stair machines to treadmills to stationary bikes, there are also machines for every muscle in your body. Some people may think that they just need to worry about their heart health by keeping their blood pressure and cholesterol down with aerobic exercise, but the fact is that they need a *full-body* workout.

At the end of the day, we use our arms and our legs to get in and out of cars, up and down the stairs using a banister, getting in and out of bed and, of course, up and down off the toilet. That's just taking care of ourselves. Those who care for *someone else,* such as an aging parent or spouse, quickly learn that they need their *full-body strength* to transport them around or even push them in a wheelchair.

I often muse about how cool it would be to have a gym made up of objects of daily living. How about a gym that had a piano to push from one end of the gym to the other? Or how about moving a recliner up and down a staircase? Or pushing a wheelchair full of concrete blocks up a ramp or doing squats lifting a desk. I used to carry a metal briefcase to work every day just so that I could do bicep curls while walking across the office parking lot from my car to the front door of the office. If I had a gym, I think it would have a row of increasingly heavier briefcases instead of barbells. (PS If anyone opens this kind of gym, I want a royalty. You read about it here first!)

OK, I will stop here and let you yell a little. Remember, I do a lot of work for the CDC and they don't even let me use the word *exercise* because they say that people hate that word. Heaven forbid you mention the word *gym*, which scares people even more because they are afraid of people staring at them, shaming them or hitting on them. *Give me a break!* This is *your life* we are talking about.

People hit on people at bars, and people haven't stopped going to them. If I hated going to the grocery store or hated the service at restaurants, would I stop eating? I hate the airports, but I still fly. I hate traffic, but I still drive.

My biggest retort to gym haters is that there are dozens of choices. There are country club gyms and urban gyms. There are gyms just for women and warehouse gyms for muscle heads. There are fighting gyms and family gyms. There are heart-rate gyms, cross-fit gyms, and even surfboard gyms (seriously). There are expensive ones and cheap ones. There are office gyms and community gyms. There are even parks with outdoor gym equipment, so choose your kind of gym. Try different ones. Just pick one and go.

Trust me, I get it. Go ahead and tell me again how much you hate the gym and get it out of your system. Throw the book down. I don't care.

I've heard it from my family and friends for years that they don't want to spend the money. They don't like having to dress in tight clothes or clothes that show their fat or any kind of special clothes to go to the gym. They feel intimidated. They don't like to shower there. They don't like to go to the bathroom at the gym. (News flash, neither do I.) They think it is just one big laboratory full of germs sitting on every piece of equipment, which it is. Sweaty people gross them out. They don't like the smell of the gym. You name it, I've heard it, and yet I know very few people who consistently get a full-body workout in their living room at home.

Of course, it's not for a lack of home-gym equipment or home-aerobic videos. They are ubiquitous. They are on TV and DVDs and social media. (I picked up my first home-exercise machine as trash on the side of the curb, for goodness sake!) Unfortunately, putting in an hour on a treadmill in your basement or bedroom when the rest

of the family is watching TV gets old fast. I get it. Plus, a Peloton®
bike may not fit with your living room decor.

According to the Centers of Disease Control and Prevention
(CDC), only 50 percent of *all adults* over eighteen meet the aerobic
Physical Activity Guidelines. Worse is that only 21 percent meet
the guidelines for aerobic activity *and* muscle strengthening activity.
That means only one in five adults in the entire nation work on their
muscles apart from their lungs. That's totally nuts.

People often point to our healthcare and insurance system as the
responsible parties for our poor health outcomes, but the majority
of blame sits firmly on the American people. Half of the entire
population is sitting, and four out of five have invited some chips
and beer to join them on the couch.

Apart from the other brainless reasons to join a gym, the absolute
best reason to sign up is the positive peer pressure that lives there.
When you enter a gym, you enter a different dimension.

At some level, everybody at the gym is there to *trade discipline
now for a payday later.* They have plenty of other things that they *could
be* doing or would *rather be* doing. They are not bored with life and
have nothing better to do than go hang out with sweaty strangers. The
people at the gym have a goal they're working toward. It might be to
lose weight or to lift it. It actually might be to build discipline. Just being
in a place of goals will deliver a powerful mental and emotional punch.

In fact, let's redefine the word *GYM* as the *Goals You* can
Measure. Seriously, how many other places in life can you measure
your progress? How many activities allow you to measure your
improvement? Sure, you have reviews at work, and you can dust
your house and brush your teeth until visible results emerge. But
advancement is hard to tap into once you leave high school. Where
else can you go and measure your increases in ability, day in and day
out with distance and strength?

I used to have a gym in my basement. It was bad ass. It cost me
about $5,000 and had a lot of bells and whistles. I installed mirrors

on the walls and music speakers to pump me up. I even had a water cooler. I was ready to get huge. I entered a contest to win a sports car if I transformed my body. I set my goals high. Even though I was disciplined to hit the weights and the treadmill, I couldn't meet my goals. I talked to friends and I couldn't figure it out.

After I moved, I sold the equipment in my basement with the house (because I couldn't move it) and I joined a gym in my new community. Suddenly, I started to see dramatic results. I couldn't figure it out until one day I caught myself pushing myself beyond my usual quitting point. I was doing pull-ups and I was ready to drop to the floor when suddenly I caught sight of a guy nearly twice my age doing pull-ups twice as fast as me. A spark of competition ignited in me and I didn't let go of that bar. Instead I kept going, ten . . . fifteen . . . twenty . . . struggling like a middle schooler to finish my last rep. I realized that was what was happening every day, unbeknownst to me. I was competing with complete strangers. I didn't care what they thought, I just wanted to beat them in my imaginary competition.

Similarly, I will typically start walking on the treadmill and slowly punch up the arrow key a little, feeling proud about just being at the gym so early in the morning. Suddenly, someone jumps on the treadmill next to me and cranks it up. That is all I need to get serious. Not everyone is competitive, and it is not necessary to improve your health. But most of us are inspired when we see someone twice as heavy or twice as old doing twice as much as us. It helps to move us beyond our comfort zone, and suddenly results start to show up sooner.

Today, we are living in an age where shows like *The Biggest Loser* are a national TV phenomenon. People cheer for people that want to improve their health and fitness. I saw a poster that read, *Fitness is the new sexy,* and I couldn't agree more. Fitness isn't about body shape or weight. It is about health and how well your body functions. Fitness is a measure of one's ability to move, to breathe, to stretch, to flex and to contract. It is also fluid. Fitness is a life measure that can move up or down, but inside the gym it has nowhere to go but up.

Sure, there are narcissists in every gym. Sure, there are people on steroids with unhealthy goals showing off. But who cares? Seriously, I've been going to my gym every morning for five years and I don't even talk to the woman who signs me in. She doesn't know my name and I don't know hers. I don't talk to anyone. I'm not there to make friends. I'm there to bring health to my body. Period.

Of course, if you want to make friends, you will have no problem doing so. I see tons of people chatting it up in every corner. In general, people at the gym are a community that values health. It is a community of people who have decided to make sacrifices in their schedule to exercise and become fit. It has become part of their routine, part of their personal constitution. It is just what they do.

As I said earlier, morning workouts are best for me. I enjoy going to work having already accomplished something. If I end up having a horrible day and feel like I didn't get anything accomplished, at least I exercised that day.

Now, if you like a little adventure, try going to a 5K or 10K run or a triathlon or a marathon. Heck, you don't even need to sign up to see what I'm talking about. Just go there. You will encounter one of the most positive groups of people on planet Earth. They help each other. They share their food and drink. They say hello and encourage each other along the race route. If you haven't tried a race, go for it and test my theory. You will absolutely be blown away. There is something contagious about positivity, and it will affect every area of your life. These people who have fallen in love with fitness are all about sharing that love. I guarantee that you will want to be like them.

TRUE STORY

Soon after I took a new job, a coworker approached me to enter a triathlon. Understand that I had never run a 5K, let alone competed in a triathlon. I didn't even have a bike because it had been stolen years ago. Since I was the new guy at the office, I wanted to make a good impression. A friend gave me his bike and I started riding every day. One day, my colleague at work told me that her friends who were also entering the triathlon were going for a group ride. I was terrified that I would be left in the dust, but I agreed to go. *Sure enough, I was left in the dust.* I sucked so bad that I circled back to the parking lot after the first lap and drove off before anyone could see me. The next day, my colleague asked me where I had gone, and I made up some excuse. Nevertheless, I did not quit.

As slow as I expected to be on the bike (and the run), I was downright terrified of drowning during the swim portion of the triathlon. I had heard horror stories of 1,000 people rushing into the water together and people getting kicked in the head and being pinned under the water. I could barely swim two laps in the community pool (no joke) and that was without anyone in my lane. How was I going to survive in the open water? Out of pure terror, I started getting up at 5 a.m. in the pitch black and sneaking into my neighborhood outdoor pool. The pool and clubhouse were so dark I couldn't see anything. Moreover, the water was freezing. I think my fear, coupled with the chill of the water, made me swim faster.

On race day, I could still only swim down and back four times in my small neighborhood pool before gasping for air. But the adrenaline and positive energy of the entire community carried me through each leg of the race and across the finish line. My teenage son came with me to cheer me on and take pictures of this momentous event. It was a baby triathlon, called a sprint, but I assure you that I never sprinted any part of it. The race was exhausting but I finished. I still remember the absolute exhilaration of crossing the finish line. We all got a medal and went to breakfast afterward. I ordered everything on the menu.

The point of that story is to embrace exercise and to not be afraid to push your limits. Don't call it physical activity. Call it exercise and just do it. Expect it to be hard. Expect to hurt the next day. But also expect to feel exhilaration for simply doing it. Don't be afraid of it.

Treat it like a challenge. No one is going to judge you. (No one is even paying attention to you!) Everyone is going to admire you for trying. I *love* to see people who are overweight in my gym. I smile at them. I nod and convey my respect that they refuse to accept their health condition. They nod back at me, because I, too, refuse to accept *my* health condition!

Most people never try. So, just attempting a run or a walk, or simply joining a gym, or getting out of bed early (or buying a bit of spandex) is downright admirable.

The other point of that story is that I didn't belong to a gym at the time of my crazy triathlon training. I didn't have extra money to join a fancy gym, and there wasn't a cheap one close to my house. I used what was available—a sidewalk, a donated bike and a neighborhood pool—to increase my heart rate and burn calories and build strength and endurance. I can honestly say that single event was the turning point in my life regarding exercise.

Ever since I started that training regimen, I have been hooked. Sure, I have fallen off the wagon here or there, but the habit was formed and *forged*. The hooks had sunk into my brain. My metabolism and mental drive had been activated.

In case you are still not convinced that a gym is for you, and if you are thinking that you don't know anyone that goes to your local gym, let me assure you that I don't know anyone who goes to my gym either. I like that. I go there on purpose to be alone. I wear my headphones and listen to music, audio books or podcasts. I don't talk to anyone and I don't expect or want anyone to talk to me. I crave the solitude, early in the morning. I also love the anonymity because I want to grimace and grunt and sweat (like an injured animal) and not worry about what people think of me, let alone know my name. My clothes don't match, and I wear things that don't fit me. That's another benefit of working out in the morning when there are fewer people around. Truth be known, a lot of other people seem to dress with similar lack of fashion sense. Fortunately, most people are so bleary-eyed that they can't see straight, let alone evaluate each other's wardrobe. Sometimes, I don't even wash my face (sorry). I just rub the sleepy out of my eyes with a dry hand and stumble into my car. The longer I take in the kitchen or bathroom in the morning, the harder it is for me to make it to the gym. (Remember, my goal is just to *get to the gym*.)

In summary, I'm saying that you can be successful at the gym *with* friends or without any. You can find success before work or after work, after fifteen minutes or after an hour and fifteen minutes. The common element is the *decision and commitment* to end the excuses.

In the past, few office buildings had gyms, and hotel gyms were usually the size of a closet if they existed. Today, a lot of office buildings have gyms and hotels advertise their expansive gyms on the home page of their websites. They invest in state-of-the-art equipment and even give you free running shoes and workout clothes if you need them for free. Unbelievable. Even cruise ships (the definition of caloric excess) promote their massive, beautiful gyms. If you go on a cruise, you may just end up having the gym to yourself, which is awesome. Bottom line, working out has never been easier than in the twenty-first century.

These days, whenever I travel, I make it a rule that I ask about the gym before I select my hotel, and then I force myself to go to the gym every day that I stay there. It has become a badge of honor. I was in line at Starbucks one day with my colleagues on a business trip. We were all moaning about the early start-time of the meeting and someone whined that the meeting was so early, they couldn't work out. Then they turned to me and asked, "Did you work out, John?" to which my other friend replied for me, "Of course he did. He always does." Of course, I *don't always* work out when I travel, but I try to. Sure enough, on that particular day I had. Even if you only have fifteen or twenty minutes, it is always better than zero minutes. Even a fifteen-minute workout, practiced consistently, will change your brain and create a habit. That's the key. Exercise as a habit. Exercise as brainless.

When traveling for work or on vacation, I've been known to run fifteen minutes to a health club and pay a guest fee so that I can use a better gym than the one at my hotel. Once, I bought a guest membership at the Boone Pickens YMCA in Dallas while I was staying there for a three-day conference. I loved that Y. Sometimes, if you are willing to take a tour of the gym, they will give you a free day pass. It's worth it to me.

As with everything in this book, joining a gym is brainless. It is easy and painless. So just do it. Stop with the excuses and join. Until you join, you won't be able to *stop* going or *start complaining about it*. Don't overthink it. Don't analyze it. I don't care how much debt you have; cutback somewhere else. This is your health, for goodness sake! This is your body. This is your heart. This is your investment in your family and in the length of time you have to make memories together. So, march down to the gym and hand over your credit card for a nice reoccurring bill of health every month.

You don't need one of their sales reps to show you around the facility unless that's what you want. And you don't need one of their free body fat assessments with one of their personal trainers, although they can be helpful. The personal training thing is not brainless. You need to check out all of their trainers if you want a good experience, and pick one that will do more than simply watch their social media feed while you do pushups in front of them on the floor.

A few years ago, I had hit a plateau. So, I hired one of the gym's trainers. He happened to be an injured NFL player. He was doing personal training to give him something to do while he was home in Atlanta recovering. He was perfect for me because I wanted someone to kick my ass. Unfortunately, he kicked it so hard that I would go to work after each session about to throw up. He pushed me to the point where I had to close my office door and put my head between my legs to breathe, even two hours following my workout. It was insane, but he taught me tons about working out.

Remember, if you really, truly hate health clubs, gyms or fitness studios because of the smell or the mirrors or the music or the abundance of spandex, then let me offer this suggestion—deal with it. Trust me on this and you will thank me, I promise. You will get stronger. You will begin to walk or jog longer and you will start to feel so much better about yourself every day that you leave the gym. You will feel pride. You will be in the 1 percent of people who consistently show up and invest in their physical health.

So, lace up your shoes tomorrow morning and then drive your body to the front door of the gym. You weren't born yesterday. You will figure out what to do. If you can't figure something out, then just do some jumping jacks and look around at other people and copy what they are doing. Or you can always ask for help from one of the bored trainers that are typically standing around. They love that. It makes them feel amazing. Someone is asking for their advice. Could it be simpler? I don't think so. Send me a before-and-after picture of yourself *at the front door*. You can send me a body-improvement picture later if you want, but I just want to see a shot of you at the front door of your gym. If you do, I'll send you a free brainless health gift. Post it on Instagram and tag @BrainlessHealth (and tag the gym). I really want to celebrate your achievement. PS If you do it, email me your mailing address, along with the post, so I can send you your gift! Email it to johnpatton@BrainlessHealth.com

I hope you have noticed that my focus in this chapter, and the entire book, is *not* centered around weight loss. If you need to lose weight in order to get your body in a healthy state, then lose weight. In other chapters I will address healthy eating for the purpose of fueling your body with good stuff. I doubt anyone minds losing weight, but weight is not the goal. *Health is the goal*, and it just happens that losing weight is often the delightful consequence of becoming healthy.

I mention this because changing one's diet (not diet*ing*) is often one of the hardest health habits to develop. Fortunately, many of the people that I interviewed for this book reported that when they started exercising (genuinely sweating), the food part of the equation started to take care of itself. That is simply because when you really exercise you feel good-and the last thing you want to do is order a pizza after you finish a good run. Nobody has to tell you *not* to order the pizza; you just don't want to (or don't want to as much).

These days I am still a rat, but now I'm one that sniffs out protein bars, throws back a handful of nuts, blends up a smoothie or downs a vegetable drink. It's crazy, but I've become a health-rat. I eat things like kale and drink Kombucha. I never ate or drank those kinds of foods before. Now I fuel with things that will deliver energy, alertness and a new sense of self-confidence.

But more importantly, I don't want to sabotage my workouts or my health gains with crap. Sure, I still have cravings, and sure I will reward myself. I say, "Hey, I want some ice cream today," and I have some. The difference now is that I will typically choose a low sugar variety that still tastes amazing. Previously, I would overindulge because I was already feeling lethargic and defeated. I was usually exhausted and overworked or overwhelmed with child rearing, long work hours, or a stubborn winter cold and I would console myself with food. That's normal. That's typical. And that is a super slippery slope. But once I started to regularly exercise, my body adjusted. The cravings subsided to a large degree and my attitude toward food *completely changed.*

Bottom line is that when you exercise, your diet improves. Try it out for yourself and see. It's actually *beyond brainless* because it will just happen automatically.

Another thing that just happens is that you are mathematically reducing the time that you have to eat. Think about it. Are you snacking on Cheetos in the gym? Are you scooping handfuls of potato chips while you are running? You are practically shortening the time you have available in the day to consume unhealthy food. Plus, you are staying busy, and that busyness causes your brain to focus on other things besides food. Have you ever been so busy that you forgot to eat? Perhaps you were so excited working on something fun or trying to meet a deadline or having such a great time with friends, or playing in the ocean, that you forgot to eat? That's because your brain stopped thinking about food. I'm not saying that is a healthy strategy, but I'm pointing out the fact that while exercising you limit the hours that you have for unhealthy behaviors.

For the very few people who honestly don't have a gym near them or honestly can't find $10 each month to spend on a gym membership, then I suggest turning your home into your gym. Not the way I built my home gym, but rather by filling a backpack with books and going for a long walk around the block. Do sit-ups or pushups. Lift up one end of your dining room table ten times. Do the same with your bed. Run the stairs in your house or in your building. Lift a chair over your head ten times. Do air-squats. Do planks. You get the idea. Make your body work. Make it sweat. Build your strength and increase your heart rate.

There are eight million free videos on YouTube about working out at home. It's not rocket science and it doesn't have to cost a single penny. Start measuring your goals one exercise, rep, minute or pound at a time. Get on it. Period. Your body needs it and the *quality of your life* depends on it.

CHAPTER SEVEN

ANTI-AMERICAN HEALTH SECRET

AMERICA DOES NOT celebrate sleep. That's the sad truth. If we truly understood the power of sleep, then a hammock would be the symbol of success. If you are successful enough to drive a luxury car, live with a two or three-car garage and buy designer jeans, you should be kicking back and chilling at least once a week in a hammock. Snoozing in the sun on a breezy day should be the expected reward for such success.

Instead, our society shuns it. It often treats sleep as a sign of laziness. It is tolerated if you are on vacation, but let's be serious, you had better be reading a business book or *New York Times* best-selling novel in your lounge chair—or at least tell people you read one. The idea of just drinking some suds in the sun is almost anti-American.

Fueling this idea are the ubiquitous business stories about CEOs who get four hours of sleep a night. Or the big-shot entrepreneur who slept in his car and worked two jobs while he launched the hottest IPO. Those stories don't include sleep. These people somehow defy nature and we treat them like real-life superheroes.

T-shirts are often a commentary on culture, and just the other day, I saw one that read, *Sleep is overrated.* Another one I saw online said, *Sleep is for the weak,* and Caribou Coffee has a famous one that says, *Life is short. Stay awake for it.* You get it. The fact is that sleep is simply not valued or seen as an essential elixir.

According to the CDC, one in three Americans don't get enough sleep. As a result, we are hurting our bodies in a big way, which is why I am devoting a chapter to the simple topic of sleep. Again, the CDC says that "insufficient sleep has been linked to the development and management of a number of chronic diseases and conditions, including diabetes, cardiovascular disease, obesity, and depression."

Enough said. Case closed. Point made. Lack of sleep makes you sick.

Forget about the science for a moment and answer this: do you feel better or worse after a good night's sleep? *Brainless, right?* We don't need the government or the medical community to teach us the power of sleep. We like the effect of a good night's sleep, so we need to get to bed with time to benefit our bodies.

Yes, it is difficult. For goodness sake, there are the kids' science projects to do and dinner to clean up, and of course we have to catch a West Coast game or Stephen Colbert's monologue. I get it. In fact, we are often so busy and stretched beyond reason that when we get into bed, we want a little bit of entertainment for ourselves. We want to catch up on our favorite TV drama. We finally have time *for ourselves,* and so we end up staying up instead of sleeping. But we always end up hurting ourselves.

It's no different than being exhausted and depressed and turning to the ice cream carton or potato chip bag. It feels like it will help us, but in the end, it only hurts us.

But like everything I present in this book, I'm not asking you to stop watching sports or HGTV. Fortunately, we live in a technological utopia where we don't have to watch the game or the news, or a season premiere when it is live. I know people who watch the *evening* news during their *lunch* hour. Better yet, we can watch the highlights of an entire sports game in minutes. Therefore, we need to start considering those options instead and stop staying up all night to the detriment of our bodies and brains.

The human body rebels as we age. It shouts at us the next day louder than it did the year before. Ask anyone in their forties how they felt the day after staying out till 3 a.m. and you will hear them admit that it takes much longer to bounce back. I love staying out late. I love shutting places down. It makes me feel like I'm back in college, and it's a rare privilege now that I have kids. I love staying up late, yet it nearly kills me the next day. I feel like a train ran over me.

Sleep doesn't just feel good, it actually helps your brain. According to Alyssa Sparacino, writing for Health.com, sleep improves your memory. Dr. Rapoport, an associate professor at NYU Langone Medical Center, says that if you are trying to learn something, you will learn it better when you sleep. Your brain does something called *memory consolidation*. (See: http://www.health.com/health/gallery/0,,20459221,00.html)

Additionally, a study showed that college students with insufficient sleep had worse grades than those who had adequate sleep.

Sleep also helps curb inflammation. Apparently, people who get less than six hours of sleep a night have *higher blood levels of inflammatory proteins* than those who get more sleep. Amazing.

Now for the drum roll, please . . . sufficient sleep actually increases fat loss. Yep. Over 50 percent of weight loss was from fat cells among well-rested people as opposed to muscle loss among the poor sleepers. "Sleep and metabolism are controlled by the same sectors of the brain," Dr. Rapoport says. "When you are sleepy, certain hormones go up in your blood, and those same hormones drive appetite." Now you know why you get the munchies when you are up late at night.

"As a nation, we are not getting enough sleep," said Wayne Giles,

MD, dean of the University of Illinois at Chicago School of Public Health.

"Lifestyle changes such as going to bed at the same time each night, rising at the same time each morning and turning off televisions, computers and mobile devices in the bedroom, can help people get the healthy sleep they need."

That makes loads of sense. I could go on and on about negative effects of ambient light from mobile devices—or the buzzing that we have become so sensitive to that it can wake us from a deep sleep. But recently I learned that our cell phones emit something called *blue light*, which is all around us. It is emitted from the sun but also from flat-screen TVs, computers, florescent lights and mobile devices. While our eyes are pretty good at blocking UV rays from hitting our retinas at the back of our eyes, the blue light cruises straight through to the retina and can lead to macular degeneration. Think blindness. That's just the tip of the iceberg when it comes to overexposure to devices, but let's just cut to the chase and agree that you need to get into bed faster and stay there for at least seven hours. And if you sleep next to someone, there are other health benefits that you and your partner can enjoy by getting more sack-time together. (More to come on that later.)

Of course, there are a ton of people who can't go to sleep even though they desperately want to. I empathize. I used to suffer from insomnia, and it was brutal. *Sleep deprivation is what they do to prisoners and terrorists to make them talk.* It is pure torture to not be able to sleep. Unfortunately, pills should never be the first answer. Ambien and other drugs are not only common, socially accepted prescriptions, but they can cause untold disasters.

At your next cocktail party, try throwing around the word Zolpidem. It is the active ingredient in many sleep aids such as Ambien˚, Ambien CR˚, Edluar˚, and Zolpimist˚ to treat short-term insomnia. They are fully approved by the FDA; however, in 2010, approximately one third (or 20,793) of the 64,175 hospital emergency department visits involving Zolpidem resulted from overmedication, according to the Substance Abuse and Mental Health Services Administration (SAMHSA). (See: http://archive.samhsa.gov/data/2k14/DAWN150/sr150-zolpidem-2014.htm)

That means people end up taking too many pills to help them sleep. If it doesn't work, they try another one, and soon your loved one is sitting next to you in an ambulance. This is insane, but not uncommon in our prescription drug society.

I will save my rant for later, but I suggest that you try my brainless rhyme, "*A pill a day, will make you pay.*"

That's not to say that prescription drugs are bad. They can be extremely good, including pain killers and sleep aids, but they come with a cost. Of course, they make you pay through your wallet as well, but more importantly they make you pay with mild to severe side effects.

The goal of this book is *not* to get you off meds, although simple lifestyle changes can often achieve that. I'm here to prevent you from having to get on the meds in the first place or get on more meds. Many people ask their doctor for a pill, assuming they have no choice or assuming that changing their lifestyle will be too hard. Neither is the case. Tell your doc about what ails you and then ask your doc about any drug-free solutions first.

Like I said, I used to be an insomniac. What changed was my exercise regimen. I stopped doing lame exercises and started to sweat profusely. I stopped doing the popular circuit workout with eight-to-twelve reps and I started to push my body with heavier weights and more reps. By the way, it is critical to include weightlifting in any routine because as I mentioned in the last chapter, your muscle strength decreases over time and you will need your muscles even more than ever as you age. Therefore, you need to literally exhaust your limbs, stretch your muscles to the point of complete fatigue. Plus, weightlifting has longer calorie-burning effects after you finish exercising than cardio. That means your body will keep burning calories and expending energy after you take your shower. Remember, this is how you kill insomnia. Your goal is sleep, and that sleep will have a compounding health impact on your body just like compounding interest. You will wake up with more energy and be able to exercise harder and sleep better and exercise harder and sleep better, etc.

I also changed my cardio to end my insomnia. I started doing what is popularly referred to as HIIT (High Intensity Interval Training). You can look it up on the internet to learn more, but basically it involves running hard for a couple of minutes and then chilling to a light jog or walk for a short period of time and then repeating it for about twenty minutes. The key is exhaustion. Fear not, you will recover just fine, and then you will sleep like a log no matter what time of day you do it. Whatever worries you and keeps you up at night will stand no chance against solid, physical exhaustion.

Please note that working out right before a meal typically curbs your appetite as opposed to the common myth that it gives you a voracious appetite. Also, please don't exercise right before bed. Obviously, exercise increases your heart rate and pumps blood to every orifice of your body, so even if you are exhausted, you need an hour or more to chill out and let everything return to normal before you can expect to sleep. At that point your body will give up and you will crash on your bed.

I recently saw an Instagram post that said, "*The two things I hated most as a kid, I now desperately want: spankings and naps.*" I won't be addressing the spanking part, but I can definitely say that naps have become like candy to me. If there is a chance for a nap, I look forward to it like a kid looks forward to Christmas. Whenever our bodies scream out for something, such as food, water or sleep, it usually means our bodies are already in a state of physical distress. I consider it DEFCON two, on its way to one. We should not wait to let our bodies start telling us things, but when they do, we must listen.

Did you ever notice that when you get a good night's sleep your face looks better? Not just the bags under your eyes, but your entire face. The skin is tighter, and blemishes are less inflamed. It's amazing. That benefit alone should make you slap on the sleep mask and hit the sheets. Sleep masks and earplugs are another way to increase the quality and duration of sleep. You won't have ambient noise or light distracting you or keeping you from a serious slumber. I personally use white noise to drown out the house creaks and the early morning birds. It makes a world of difference.

An improved face is only the start of the benefits of sleep. *Relationships* improve when you are not tired as well. Ninety percent of the time, when my colleagues, my wife or my kids are irritable, it's a sure bet that they haven't slept well. I can say that because I am more irritable when I am tired. I also *worry more* when I am sleep deprived. When I awake after a good sleep, my previous worries typically have diminished or disappeared. Try it the next time you are worried. Tell yourself that you are going to address the issue as soon as you wake up. Then drop it and see what happens in the morning. Likely, your worries will seem less ominous.

HALT

Here's a bonus. A great, brainless acronym for preventing bad decisions is HALT. It stands for Hungry, Angry, Lonely or Tired. That simple acronym is designed to cause you to *halt* before starting an argument, worrying or making any weighty life decisions if you are experiencing one or more of those four conditions. I think they all negatively affect decision-making, but for me, the most acute is tiredness. The brain simply cannot process information when it wants to shut down.

At the end of the day, sleep is a habit, and we sometimes attach other habits to it, such as nighttime rituals. Of course, you have heard about drinking milk before bed to help you sleep. I knew a man who drank a Coors Light right before bed. (It had to be Coors Light.) I don't do that personally, so I can't speak to its effectiveness, but a lot of people shower before bed, write in a journal or read. Some check their email (insane!) and others make to-do lists.

I personally advocate sex before bed for the many sleep benefits, of course. But my point is that our habits, good or bad, could be getting in the way of sleep. Feel free to take an inventory of your sleep-prep habits and see if they are giving you the most *zzzz's* for your time on the pillow. At the very least, get into bed at a reasonable time *and give your body the opportunity* to sleep and recharge.

I'd be remiss to let you think that your attention to sleep is somehow *optional*. Don't be mistaken. Nothing in this book is optional if your goal is optimal health for life. There are plenty of things like eating more vegetables that would be great to do, but they are not brainless. They require research on what to buy, how to prepare them, and when to eat them.

Getting enough sleep, however, can literally be a life-or-death matter and is simple to execute. Set your alarm if you must. Tell your partner that you are going to start to go to bed at a certain time. If they want to watch TV with you or do anything else, then they need to plan for it before you doze off.

The Association for the Advancement of Automotive Medicine estimates that one in twenty-five adults report that they have fallen asleep while driving *within the last thirty days! * Hello? That's nuts. That's 13 million American's snoozing at the wheel every month. They estimate that over 6,000 fatalities are caused by drowsy driving *every year.* That's 6,000 aunts and uncles and parents and teens dead today because people are not sleeping enough. *Even if you aren't the one asleep at the wheel, you better be wide awake to avoid those who are snoozing.*

So, get to bed. Period. I'm a big fan of the "early to bed, early to rise" adage. It may seem valiant to burn the candle at both ends, but in the end, you just end up getting burned.

VACATIONS ARE PART OF THE SLEEP EQUATION

Why are vacationing and sleep connected? Because part of *vacationing* involves sleeping. Whether you are sightseeing in Italy, sitting by the beach or simply enjoying a staycation, it usually includes sleeping in, if not outright napping during the day. Typically, it includes a reduction in stress and some yummy food, which both help to induce sleep. While alcohol can also be part of vacations, too much can inhibit sleep despite the fact that you pass out and think that you are getting wholesome rest. You are of course sleeping, but the quality of the sleep is significantly subpar, so please do not think that getting drunk is somehow a smart sleep-aid.

The bottom line is we need vacations. They help the body and the mind and our relationships.

Unfortunately, in 2015, Americans hit an all-time high (or low, if you will) for not taking all of their vacation time. In fact, according to Allianz Global Assistance, 56 percent of Americans did not vacation last year. Zero sun and sand. Zero ski sloping. Zero Griswold family vacation. That's over 130 million Americans that did not vacation whatsoever.

Lynn Parramore, in an article for Reuters, recalls that "John Maynard Keynes, one of the founders of modern economics, made a famous prediction that by 2030, advanced societies would be wealthy enough that leisure time, rather than work, would characterize national lifestyles."

Sorry, Mr. Keynes, that's not happening. Instead of rewarding our work success with leisure, we just work more.

Vacations are seen similarly to a lot of people's overall view of sleep. If sleep is a sign of weakness, *then vacations are sometimes seen as a sign of laziness.* As I wrote earlier, some people expect you to come back from a vacation with an activity report—stories about mountains climbed, waves surfed, or museums visited. Of course, for many people, active vacations that include hikes and bikes and sights are as restful to the soul as a nap in Naples, and hopefully the kind of friends you have will support you even if you simply drank mimosas, read magazines and napped in your chair every day. To each his own if renewal is part of the recipe.

In fact, business interview coaches will tell you never to ask about how much vacation you will receive as part of your first interview. Truth is, we should. We should say, "I need to know how much this company values vacation." Furthermore, ask if you are expected to answer emails while you are away. Or are you expected to answer office calls from the beach?

Sadly, it's not just pressure from the workplace staff or culture. It is often a byproduct of our actual workload. The American worker is swamped and can't seem to either find or justify the time to take time off. I have often lamented that I get punished by my email for going on vacation. In addition to adding a mountain of work to my list when I return, things fall through the cracks and opportunities get missed when replies aren't sent. Even the best efforts at posting an *out of office* message typically goes unheeded by 90 percent of the people in my experience. The mantra isn't "I'll contact him when he gets back," but rather "I'll email him now and he can *read it* when he gets back," which just puts a greater burden on the vacationer. Additionally, vacations can be full of hard work. You have heard (or said) the words yourself: "I need a vacation from my vacation." That's just honesty. Saving money, researching, planning and executing a vacation, especially a family vacation with lots of individual agendas and special considerations, is a real project. Add to that a few hundred miles of highway construction or delayed flights or overbooked hotels, and it is no wonder a lot of us pass on the idea of a vacation.

This is all very backward. According to Lolly Daska writing for *Inc. Magazine* in 2016, three out of five Americans that do go on vacation admit to working during it.

A number of studies support the relationship between vacation (or the lack thereof) and the risk for heart disease *and death.*

The Multiple Risk Factor Intervention Trial for the Prevention of Coronary Heart Disease, sponsored by the National Institutes of Health's Heart, Lung, and Blood Institute, followed 12,000 men over a nine-year period that had a high risk for coronary heart disease. The study found that men who took frequent annual vacations were 21 percent less likely to die from any cause and were 32 percent less likely to die from heart disease.

The landmark Framingham Heart Study, the largest and longest-running study of cardiovascular disease, revealed that men who didn't take a vacation for several years were 30 percent more likely to have heart attacks compared to men who took time off. And women who took a vacation only once every six years or less were almost eight times more likely to develop coronary heart disease or have a heart attack compared to women who vacationed at least twice a year.

At some of America's best companies, CEOs are finally realizing the health benefits of vacations when it comes to reducing absenteeism, decreasing medical claims and increasing employee retention. I recently read about one CEO who actually walks cubicle to cubicle to ask each employee if they are burning all of their vacation days as expected by the company. That's a truly brilliant move.

If you ever want to learn more on the subject, or just want to impress your HR director, try Googling *"Health Benefits of Vacation"* and you will find countless erudite articles on the subject. I'm not making this stuff up. It's real, and it is *really important* that you take it seriously for your own health.

Working too much has also been linked to mental health problems and a decrease in the quality of work produced. Amazingly, there is research that shows that the highest-performing employees take the *most* time off work (See: https://curiosity.com/topics/to-boost-your-performance-at-work-do-things-other-than-work-curiosity/). In fact, my wife's company joined hundreds of other companies that have instituted unlimited vacation. To some employers, that might sound crazy, but the fact is that many companies are focusing on simply getting the work done versus logging a bunch of hours behind a desk. They realize that when people are limited to a few weeks of vacation, they can spend work hours trying to *rig the system* by maximizing their allotted sick leave (even when they aren't sick) or taking long lunch hours to get the mundane tasks of life accomplished. Consequently, productivity suffers.

Additionally, a recent study by GlassDoor found that the biggest reason people don't take vacation is fear over job security. They are worried that someone will take over their work when they're absent and management will realize that the company operated fine without them. Worst of all, *Forbes* reported that most employees reported that their companies simply don't encourage taking vacations. (See: https://www.forbes.com/sites/neilhowe/2017/06/30/why-americas-overstressed-workers-wont-take-a-break/#328fdae0491f)

Of course, there's always the added factor of money. Vacationing can be expensive. The median household income in the United States still hasn't bounced back from the 2007 recession, and the nation's lowest-wage workers get the least paid vacation time.

So how does an overworked, underpaid, insecure employee manage to get a little R&R? In an article in the *Harvard Business Review*, business owner and time-management coach Elizabeth Grace Saunders advocates something that's brilliant in its simplicity—microvacations.

STOP, DROP, BREATHE

Saunders defines microvacations as periods away from work that require you to use a day (or even half a day) of vacation time. Their short duration comes with a load of benefits. You don't have to arrange for someone to handle your work; you won't come back to a mountain of emails; and you can take a lot of microvacations, for the price of one. They can also help avoid burnout. Plus, if your workplace culture discourages long vacations, short stints might be an easier sell to your boss and noticed less by your colleagues.

Here's a simple example: The next time you're feeling the squeeze of your workload, check your calendar and arrange for a single vacation day on an upcoming Friday. Why Friday? It's close to a weekend, which will give you three days off in a row, and the office workload on Fridays can sometimes be lighter, depending where you work. You could take a Monday off, but because many people wait until Monday to start projects or send important emails, the Tuesday you get back could be a doozy. Find a location where you've never been that's a few hours away and get there by Thursday night. Boom! You've got nearly three full days to kick back and recharge your batteries. It might be a mountain lodge or a tent by a creek. It might be a nearby city full of stores that you don't have in your town, or a city with a stage theater, opera or concert venue. I know a lot of people who will drive to a nearby city to see their favorite musician perform whose tour doesn't come to their town. Some of my friends prefer staying in a bed and breakfast or renting a house. Whatever floats your boat and won't break the bank can be the perfect holiday.

But the true brilliance of microvacations might just be the fact that they don't require that you go anywhere at all. Often, working long hours results in sacrifices in other areas, such as friendships, home upkeep, or the little chores and errands. You're well within your rights to take a day to paint the den or have lunch with your kid at school. Remember, vacation days are yours to use, and you define the vacation. If your job allows it, you could even take a half-day to have a long lunch with an old friend or catch a matinee at the movies.

ALL VACATIONS ARE NOT EQUAL

We all remember truly amazing vacations. We recall the food, the sunshine, the book we read, the museum, the tour, the hotel splendor or even the pillows. We remember sleeping in or greeting the morning with beach yoga or a run. They define the word *vacation*.

Conversely, when some people say they are going on vacation, they really mean they're going to visit the in-laws or the grandparents or Aunt Betty. Don't get me wrong; if visiting family defines a great vacation for you, then congratulations. Do it. But for many, visiting family can be stressful. Regardless of the level of love or stress, it is rare that visiting family offers the same healthful detachment that other kinds of vacations can provide. That's simply the nature of the beast. As good as Mom's cooking might be, she's not going to serve you like a waiter will. She's not going to make your bed every day (at least I hope not) and you aren't going to be able to just stop talking and start daydreaming out the window, without everyone wondering what is wrong.

Similarly, vacations with the kids are not always the most relaxing either. Therefore, I would suggest that you distinguish them from other vacation types. Some people call them *family vacations*, and that is a decent distinction. Most people can recount the *baby vacations* when they couldn't take their eyes off junior lest he drown in the pool, fall down the stairs or get a sunburn. From adolescence to hormonal mood swings, to setting curfews, to simply realizing how expensive dining out can be with teenagers, a family vacation can end up costing more than expected and afford little chance for bedroom intimacy—unless you pay for the kids to have their own room or are extremely quiet.

Typically, the most healthful aspects of family vacations are the memories that they create. Even if they aren't restful at the time, sweet memories of snorkeling or ski lessons can literally create healthful bliss. In fact, the mind has a way of remembering the best parts of life and forgetting the less-than-great times. This is often the case with family vacations.

The point of dissecting one's definition of vacation is to make sure you are not short-changing your body and mind from truly rejuvenating.

If cost is a concern, run away to the nearest city and stay in a hotel for just a night or two. Or just hit the local resort spa in your town for the day, followed by a nice dinner so you don't have to do the dishes. Whatever you can afford is fine. You certainly don't want your piece of relaxation to stress you out financially. Just make sure you control your circumstances. If you want to, simply stay in bed, sleep in and binge on TV shows. The goal is simply to make the effort to carve out a path that takes your mind and body to a truly happy place on a regular basis.

I had a friend who said that she needed a vacation every quarter. I thought that was excessive until I considered that it is only four breaks a year. Kids get more than four holidays in nine months of school, which is far less stressful than holding down a job, raising a family and paying the bills. A vacation could be simply extending a holiday weekend two more days and suddenly you have a five-day vacation.

There is yet another often overlooked aspect of vacations. Most of the attention is placed on the actual dates of a vacation, but there are real mental health benefits associated with *looking forward* to a vacation. It is like anticipating a holiday like Christmas or Halloween when we were kids. I remember making paper chains and cutting off a loop every day. It was awesome. I couldn't wait for the fun. Vacations can be the same way. We might start shopping for specific clothes in anticipation of its arrival. We might search the internet for cool things to see or do when we arrive at our destination. One of my friends goes so far as to research the local cuisine and make dinner reservations for every night that he's away. I'm sure plenty of people can attest that sometimes the anticipation ends up being better than the actual trip.

WORK VACATIONS

For those who travel for work, I suggest finding ways to integrate a microvacation. I try to do this when possible. As I mentioned earlier, I usually make sure the hotel has a fitness facility and plan a great workout where I can sweat and groan without any worry about running into someone I know. Sometimes the hotel will have a steam or dry sauna, and I always take advantage. Even if my meetings start early, I will get up early for a trip to the sauna. One time, I was so relaxed for a meeting a colleague asked if I was feeling alright. Isn't it funny that something can appear to be wrong with us when we feel great? It's likely because people don't see us in that state of relaxation enough.

One of my favorite work-travel activities is jogging around the city I am visiting. I recently ran all over historic Philadelphia, past Independence Hall, the Liberty Bell and City Hall. The last time I was in California, I ran down to the Santa Monica Pier. Nothing was open at 7 a.m. but the stillness of this iconic beach playland; the early morning light was spectacular. Of course, San Francisco's hills provide the perfect combination of a truly ass-kicking workout with eye-popping views and cool temperatures. And for me, nothing beats a run around Central Park in New York City. It's so massive that I see different things every time.

Since I am a serious foodie and a sucker for aesthetics, I search the web for cool places to go for dinner or drinks. As a result, I have found the best hole-in-the wall restaurants and speak-easy bars. I'll spend an evening after a day of business meetings, reclining by a 300-year-old fireplace in Aaron Burr's New York horse stable, or tucked inside a booth at the hottest W hotel listening to a DJ spinning tunes in the lobby. Rooftops are my favorite, and so I Google them every time I travel. With these little tactics you can also impress your traveling companions by either inviting them to join you or simply telling them about your discoveries the next morning. Of course, simply retiring to your room and ordering room service can also be a nice way to *vacationize* a business trip.

One of my favorite ways to turn business travel into a vacation is to ask a friend or family member to join me before my meetings begin or after they are over. If possible, I plan my travel at the beginning or end of the week so that I can tack on the weekend before or after my conference or meetings. Since travel can often be one of the most expensive parts of any vacation, having your company pay for your travel reduces your expenses considerably.

Nearly every time I travel to New York, I ask my wife along. She can't always get away, but I keep asking. Besides New York, we've visited California, Colorado, Arizona and Alaska. One of the most special trips of my life was visiting the Grand Canyon with my daughter during her junior year of college. I finished up my business meetings in Phoenix on a Thursday, met her at the airport, rented a convertible and drove to the Grand Canyon through Sedona. The scenery was spectacular, but it could not hold a candle to our conversations and the memories we made together. She got married just one year later, and that trip will likely be the last time we will ever have a solo father-daughter vacation.

At very least, a business trip should serve to find out if you ever want to come back to your destination for a real vacation. I've been to rural Louisiana, industrial Wisconsin and suburban Florida. All had redeeming qualities that would merit a return trip with my family or my wife. I've also been to beaches in California and Florida that I would never want to waste my time or money visiting on a vacation. So, the next time the office pays for your travel, try and find out if it's worth returning to when you are the one paying.

So how *do* you make vacations brainless? Good question. The answer is *your calendar*. This isn't a tip; *it is a habit* that needs to become as common as making a New Year's resolution.

Every New Year's Eve, or New Year's Day, grab your calendar. Treat this activity exactly like a doctor's appointment. Put your vacations on the calendar. *Don't roll your eyes!* I can hear you complaining about your inability to forecast so far in advance, but that is the precise reason that you must put it on the calendar. Our inability to foresee the future is why our vacations get squeezed out. We say that we will go somewhere in June, but then June comes and we haven't saved enough money or the we aren't feeling comfortable in our swimsuit, etc. But if it is on the calendar and the hotel has been reserved, we are going. We will look forward to it and we will prepare and be ready for it. Most of all, our work will not swallow it up. I have had many great intentions, only to have my colleagues schedule meetings when I had hoped to get away. *Hoping* is different than *having. Having it* on the calendar makes all the difference. And if you are flying, you better book those tickets well in advance or you will be paying double.

Write down the names of cities or parts of the world you would like to visit. Maybe you have a big event every year at the same time and you know that you could probably use a staycation afterwards to recover. Great. Put it on the calendar. Maybe you like to hit the beach before spring breakers descend or depart. Good. Put it on the calendar. Maybe your tenth anniversary is in October and you have been planning on going to Paris. Super. Put it on the calendar. Lock it in.

This process helps to make the actual *taking* of a vacation brainless because when things are on the calendar, we automatically plan *for* them and we plan *around* them. One of the biggest reasons that people don't take vacations is that life crowds them out. Rarely will you look at your calendar and declare that you have no commitments. If it isn't a business trip, it will be some child's sports commitment. It might be as simple as a Fourth of July neighborhood BBQ or a nephew's birthday. Something will likely prevent you from getting away.

Moreover, for those who control their work schedule, you can plan your meetings around certain dates or simply request time off well in advance so that it doesn't come as a surprise to the rest of your team or boss.

As mentioned, putting vacations on the calendar allows you to plan *for* them. That might mean getting in shape for the beach or the ski slopes. One of my friends was going skiing and knew that he needed to strengthen his lower back for protection before hitting the slopes. He was able to start training four months in advance because it was *already* on his calendar.

Probably the best reason to put vacations on the calendar is to help *save* for them. Saving is hard for most people to do in general, and vacations are often one of the biggest reasons that people go in debt or simply don't go at all. *A vacation that puts you in long-term debt is not a vacation. It's stupid.*

Having said that, planning for a vacation can improve your ability to save money. The key is to reallocate money you would spend on coffee or a newspaper or a new dining room table, and transfer it to your vacation fund.

You will be blown away at how fast your vacation nest egg will add up. I'm not just advocating financial savings. I'm talking about *vacation* savings. There is something nearly painless about saving for a vacation. If you need to cut out pictures of the beach or a foreign place you want to visit, go ahead. Stick them where you are most tempted to spend the money you want to be saving. I will tape a picture in my car to remind me to avoid the car wash and do it myself in my driveway to save money. Crazy simple stuff. You might not save the entire amount needed for your vacation, but it will take a huge bite out of your expenses. I've heard of some couples and families saving to pay for souvenirs or for a fancy dinner at the beach or for an activity like jet skiing or parasailing. We can all save enough for at least a part of the vacation.

The key is to *transfer* the money. Don't simply decide not to eat out. Transfer the money you would spend at a typical restaurant to your vacation fund. Then order a pizza or eat leftovers. It all starts with understanding that *a vacation is not a luxury*. It is just as important as getting braces for the kids or getting your annual physical exam. Keep that perspective and you will be less prone to steal from yourself by raiding your own vacation savings. So, get started. Grab the calendar, pick some places and start saving.

CHAPTER EIGHT

FASTER FOOD

MCDONALD'S USHERED IN the era of fast food, but it has had a lot of helpers. In addition to the dizzying number of copycat quick-serve eateries, the microwave arrived along with freeze-dried foods, cooked meals and everything in between. Then there was the dawn of thirty-minute pizza delivery. Fast and furious food consumption has become a part of most people's busy lives to some extent or another. I recently talked to a Hooters executive who reported that their to-go sector has jumped 50 percent compared to only 4 percent growth of in-store sales. Many places have mobile apps that let us order our coffee or food ahead of our arrival to avoid waiting in line. (Lines are so yesterday.) Fast food simply doesn't seem fast enough.

Now, we all know that fast food tastes fantastic, but we also know that a steady diet of fast food is simply not good for us. Period. But if the reason you eat fastfood is because you are on the go and need food that is fast, or simply because you crave the irresistible convenience of the drive-thru with a minivan full of car seats, I understand your plight. I've been there. Fortunately, we have options to increase the speed of our food and our convenience at the same time. In other words, you can have even *faster food* without sacrificing your health.

I recently had this conversation with a top television news producer who was complaining that he *had* to eat fast food because of the demands of his job. He was on the run following breaking news stories and so he *was forced* to eat unhealthy fast food despite knowing better. I heard the same from a New York City police officer. The cop said he gained fifty pounds after he joined the force because he was always having to grab something quick and that he often had to work nights when healthy food outlets were closed. McDonald's and Taco Bell were the only places that were open.

Please stop the madness. Healthy food choices have been around since the beginning of time, and just because we like the convenience of pre-cooked food doesn't mean that we are forced to eat it. Fast food entered our lexicon in the 1950s. Prior to that, fast food used to be defined as stirring the pot quickly. Since then, culture has manufactured less and less healthy options over time. We've had to *work* to introduce unhealth into our food system. Salads aren't a new invention just because they finally made it onto McDonald's menu. Healthy eating was once the rule and it didn't always involve hours of preparation or waiting.

When I tell my friends how to solve their fast-food excuses they are speechless. I tell them that if they want healthy food that is faster than fast food and more convenient than any drive-thru, then they needed to start eating protein bars and shakes. Wait! I know what you are thinking. *Yuk. A bar is not a meal. I've tried them and they are disgusting.* I get it.

Back in the day, that was the case. Protein bars tasted and looked horrible. But today, they're delicious. You can find bars of every flavor, from coconut to lemon to chocolate to coffee. There are ones made of solid protein and ones that are low on protein and full of carbs and tons of sugar. You absolutely must read the labels because not all bars are created equal, but as far as *faster food,* you can't get anything faster than unwrapping a wrapper or unscrewing a bottle top. I keep bars in the glove box of my car and in my briefcase. They are perfect to eat while watching kids' baseball practice and certainly better than a pack of M&Ms from the concession stand. I eat healthy bars on the plane or in an Uber. Honestly, I think they're a modern wonder of the twenty-first-century diet. If only people would try them. Don't hate on them because you tried one that you didn't like, and don't eschew them because of the list of crazy ingredients. I'm not recommending them as a nutritional alternative to healthy food. Rather, I simply recommend them over candy and Big Macs. Fortunately, there's no need to go to a health store or some fitness warehouse to get them. I guarantee that your local grocery store has at least fifty varieties along with protein powders, pre-workout and recovery drinks. It's amazing to me. Finally, the performance foods of elite athletes and Hollywood stars have come to main street grocery stores.

That is really all that you need to know. Keep it brainless. Go to the grocery store and get some protein powder and start making your own smoothies with a blender. You don't need to get any special equipment and you don't need any make-in-advance recipes. I put ice and water in a blender, add a scoop of protein powder and some fruit and I'm in business. Sometimes, I throw in some peanut butter, lemon juice, or beet juice. Toss a bar in your bag and the shake in a coffee mug travel cup. It's not going to magically give you a bikini body, but it will likely kill your cravings and help you shed a few pounds. You will be blown away at how quickly your body will adjust (and benefit) from fast food to even faster food.

As I said, remember that some of those bars and drinks are loaded with sugar and chemicals. You can check out my Instagram account @SugarFixChallenge to see some of the things I post that are disguised as fast-healthy but are far from it. Part of being brainless means that you automatically look at labels. That should always happen without even thinking. I call it *Brainless Back*! Look at the back of the box, bottle or bag of everything you buy!

We've all heard the phrase *you are what you eat*. In other words, you will start looking like the food you eat. I should know. I did. I used to go to my favorite bagel joint every single morning for years. I gained over twenty pounds in no time, looking exactly like the bagels I was eating (cinnamon crunch with maple cream cheese), and yet I justified it. I was stressed. I was working incredible hours. It was my only pleasure. It helped me get my day started. Plus, it was just one bagel.

Truth is, I didn't care about my weight. I only cared about getting out of bed in the morning and getting to a cold warehouse where I worked alone for sixteen hours a day. It sucked, and the reason I tell you that is because I want you to understand that I know what it is like to use food as a friend or companion or consolation for a tough job or a cold morning.

Years later, with a daughter getting married and a beach vacation approaching, I had whittled my body down to an enviable new shape that I wished I had been able to enjoy for the previous decade. I wished I had turned to something else to motivate me on all those early mornings. I wish I had turned to the gym or the juice bar. Given my current perspective on health, I can only wonder how much more successful I would have been in every aspect of life if I had hit the gym each morning instead of the bagel shop.

Now, for everyone who is still shaking their head at the idea of eating a protein bar or drinking a shake, allow me to remind you that there are millions of subscription-based, fully prepared (or prepped) meal companies that will deliver healthy meals to your door seven days a week. I've tried a few and they are great, from Blue Apron to Hello Fresh. And although I initially thought that they were too expensive, I saved money by not going to the grocery store and wasting money on impulse purchases I didn't need. Of course, if you like going to the store, go for it, but don't rule these companies out because of the monthly price tag. Plus, they can be tons of fun to prepare with your spouse or kids or friends. I love to cook, and when all of the ingredients arrive in measured amounts, it's much easier and saves me from buying a bottle of cumin or cilantro flakes.

If you still need faster food, there are meals that just need heating, and there are even healthy smoothies that arrive in cups ready to stash in your fridge and ready to grab before you head out the door. *Excuses are a thing of the past.* There is not any barrier to health that hasn't been overcome today.

GARBAGE IN, GARBAGE OUT

What computer programmers coined years ago is true for food and fitness—"garbage in, garbage out." Nothing could be more poignantly concise.

A few years ago, my wife and I were sitting on the famous Lincoln Road in Miami. We were ordering typical beach cocktails and being served by a complete Adonis of a waiter. The guy showed every ripple of his chiseled physique. I asked him his secret and was expecting this obvious party boy in the heart of Miami's heat to say that he did 100 crunches every night before bed. But he didn't.

Instead, he said that he worked out in the gym every day and only had one cheat day a MONTH. He ate ONE *slice* of pizza or ONE burger every MONTH. He said that he *never* drank alcohol. I couldn't comprehend the idea of twelve burgers a year or only a dozen slices of pizza. No judgement, it just isn't for me. My palate is more important than my pecs, but my point in telling that story is that the waiter's body reflected what it was being fed.

Fortunately, health has happy mediums for everyone. If you aren't aspiring to be on the cover of a fitness magazine, you can still be the fittest person in your office and grab a beer with your boss. You can go to the gym and still eat French fries with your kids.

I admire the discipline that it takes to have 8 percent body fat, just like I admire those who ascend Mt. Everest, but I'm just not ready to orient my lifestyle in that direction because those are not *my goals.* That is the key. *Goal discovery.* I can (and have) shared many reasons why I think you should demand a healthy life, but at the end of the day, you must discover what is going to faithfully fuel *your* health goals. Like I said in chapter two, *what is your why?*

I've talked to hundreds of people while writing this book, and every time I bring up the *topic of fast food*, people universally plead guilty to their guilty pleasure. No one defends fast food. That is because there is zero upside to fast food apart from being incredibly delicious. Even some of the salads are laden with calories. Ask for the nutrition facts and you will be amazed.

As I have written before, we are living in a great time. The grocery stores and the convenience stores and *even gas stations* carry protein bars and protein drinks now. Whenever I travel to a city on business, I go into a drug store by the hotel and grab a couple of protein drinks and then I put them on ice in my hotel room ice bucket. When I get up in the morning, I have time to exercise because my breakfast is already prepared and waiting in the fridge or in a hotel bucket of ice. I save tons of time.

I can still hear the groans of all of you who love a hot breakfast of pancakes or waffles. No one is telling you not to have them! No one loves that more than me. I start to salivate just reading the words *pecan pancake* on the menu. But indulging in unhealthy foods needs to be *your choice,* not your *circumstances* or the hands on the clock. That's the bottom line. No one is a victim, and no one should hold their body hostage because of their schedule.

And remember, if you hate protein bars, then you can always pack some celery sticks with peanut butter or carrot sticks, or rice cakes, or beef jerky, or slices of Ezekiel bread. Those things are not as packed with protein as a high quality energy bar, but at least they should keep you from detouring to a drive-thru.

THE COST MYTH OF HEALTHY EATING

I can't ignore the perpetuation of the ridiculous—and false—argument that only the rich can eat healthy. Food deserts are real. Low access to fresh produce is real, and yes, a salad sometimes costs more at a fast-food joint than a burger and fries. We must do more to address these societal issues, but in the meantime, those facts and the lack of higher wages cannot prevail as forgone conclusions or excuses for ill-health.

If you really want cheap food, go and grab a head of lettuce for 99 cents and make a salad. In fact, grab a bag of broccoli for $2.99 and a pre-chopped bag of grilled chicken for $3.99 and a bottle of salad dressing for $1.29 and voila! You have *four complete meals* for just over $2 each (topped off with a delicious, icy glass of H2O.) I can feed a family of four for less than any dollar menu, anywhere, any time while imparting health to the family. Over time, a salad will actually become more delicious than a tray full of burgers and fries. Your taste buds, stomach and brain adjust. It's awesome but it takes time.

If we help people get healthy, their new health will help them get better jobs, earn more money, raise healthy kids and live healthier lives. That's a fact. I don't care who you are or where you live or what kind of job you have or don't have. If you are not healthy, you will have a super hard time climbing the next rung of economic opportunity.

As I have said repeatedly, go ahead and have your drive-thru mega-meal from time to time. It's not a sin. It's not the devil, but don't tell me you can't afford anything else or that other people have no choice. Life is all about choices, and success comes from making *wise choices*. Period.

My teenaged stepdaughter shares my conviction. "The grocery store always has amazing, low-cost deals on fruit and vegetables," she recently said. She referenced twenty-five-cent oranges and manager specials on beans, carrots and squash. That's because her mom buys them. I personally never knew what a *manager special* was until I met my wife, Antuanette. It's the discount they put on things about to expire. They are amazing deals and we buy them all the time.

When I was a kid, we were far from rich, so we ate casseroles. Hello?! Remember that word? A casserole could almost feed the neighborhood for five bucks. How about the age-old crock-pot? Remember that? Same idea and super yummy. I grew up with saucy mystery meat on top of toast. It worked. I lived to write about it. It didn't make me an obese kid, I didn't develop Type 2 diabetes and I also didn't starve.

Some people like to tell me that low wage earners don't know how to cook. That's another bad and insulting argument that is perpetuated to the detriment of society. It is infuriating because even low-income people have cellphones, and cellphones come with YouTube and YouTube comes with step-by-step cooking lessons for every imaginable food, meal and literacy level.

I make enemies when I disagree with the assumption that eating healthy isn't an option for low-income families because it is so expensive. Sure it is hard, but not impossible, especially when it is a matter of life and death.

Repeat after me: *Eating crap is economically agnostic.* It is a choice for rich and poor alike. Few people in America are going to starve. In fact, if you look at the people living in food deserts (places without fresh fruits and vegetables), you find plenty of obese people. They are not starving, but they are malnourished. So are lawyers and doctors and movie stars. Eating healthy does not *have to* cost more. Whole Foods is not the only grocery store that sells healthy food. Every grocery store has healthy food, and every one of them has sales, BOGO, discount brands, or discontinued items.

Yes, it is horribly hard to buy fresh fruits and vegetables if you have to take three public busses to get to a grocery store, but to assume that the only alternative is to eat McDonald's or rotisserie hot dogs at the gas station is demeaning to those who face those challenges. We must help them. We must get creative. This book is not about pulling yourself up by your bootstraps; it is about ending the excuses.

When you go to Third World countries, people don't have excuses because they don't have options. They often eat healthy because they don't have unhealthy options. They walk for miles on dirt roads or dig up their food by hand in community gardens or trade fresh fruit with someone who has fresh vegetables. They pick up groceries near their work instead of near their house. Yes, it is unfair. Yes, it is hard, but it is their physical existence that we are talking about. If anything is worth working hard for, it is the breath in our lungs and the beat of our hearts. Let's identify the inequities but focus on the solutions without giving anyone an excuse. We need a zero-tolerance attitude toward a daily diet of unhealth. Period.

No one is forcing anyone to buy fast food or harmful food. Residents of public housing and suburban soccer moms are both putting themselves at risk if they repeatedly do so. Nothing makes me crazier than watching people who have education, money, transportation and access to healthy foods choose to eat crap. It is not always about those social determinants of health. It is a matter of knowing what is at stake. It is about counting the cost in the long run. It is about turning away from unhealthy choices even if a healthy choice isn't available. Just because I don't have orange juice in the fridge doesn't mean I'm justified to drink a beer for breakfast. It sucks that it is hard, but dealing with disease is far harder.

It's hard when you are poor, but it is also hard when you are wealthy and travel constantly for work or are divorced or are obsessed about keeping up with the Joneses. Rich and poor make equally damaging choices when they order another pizza or pour another cocktail. It's up to everyone to make the choice between future health or future hardship.

VITAMINS, PILLS AND POTIONS

Another aspect to the adage *you are what you eat* is the supplement and vitamin world. I'm certainly not an authority, but I use them every day. While I haven't found a multi-vitamin that doesn't upset my stomach, I take Vitamin C chewable tablets every day. Vitamin C is inexpensive and well documented to help your immune system. I keep them on hand, and when the weather fluctuates, or I start traveling a lot, I pop them like Pez®.

Zinc is another tablet that I employ when I feel the need to divert a cold. Zicam® is my chewable of choice, but it doesn't matter what you take. I even take those EmergenC® and AirBorne® tablets before bed from time to time. It might simply be the placebo effect, but it seems to help me keep from getting sick or even *thinking* I'm sick.

Typically, when we *feel* sick or under the weather, tired, anxious, weak or simply wiped out, then we often stop exercising and turn to unhealthy food. While we should always listen to our body and head to the doctor, sometimes the first feelings of illness send us into a spiral of unhealthy choices.

How many times have I reached for the Cheetos®, the chocolate pretzels, a beer or the ice cream carton when I'm feeling under the weather? It's just where I go when I'm not feeling good physically or emotionally. Certain foods release endorphins and dopamine and other chemicals in our brains that indeed make us feel better. We like to avoid pain and suffering. It's called *comfort food* for a reason.

Again, I am all for comfort, and I don't promote discomfort. We must ask ourselves how long the comfort agent will comfort us and what it will deliver for us long term. Typically, the comfort is temporary, and the discomfort comes calling soon after and sticks around. Whether it is a belly ache or a headache, it will likely last longer than the temporary food high that we enjoyed. This is especially true when it manifests as body fat that will take months or years to lose. We must find different ways to comfort ourselves.

The brain tells us to partake of the yummy, unhealthy foods when we are not feeling well. That's why we have to develop brainless tactics that go into effect without engaging our brain. When you are in a positive, healthy, solid state of mind, try to remind yourself how good you feel. Stop and notice what is going on. Take a deep breath. Look in the mirror. Suck in your stomach and admire how much you like the reflection. Remind yourself that you don't want to take any steps backward.

When we feel good physically and emotionally, then we will eat a reasonable portion of food and then push away from the table. We will enjoy the taste of the food instead of chasing the sugar hit from unhealthy foods.

Alcohol is especially suited to this application. If we are drinking to drown out sorrows, then we are only hurting ourselves, and the sorrows compound and are never extinguished. Rather, when you can enjoy a drink or two and then get back to life, you will greatly reduce the alcohol-related, ill-health effects associated with binge drinking and alcohol abuse. PS Alcohol is one of the greatest contributors to adult obesity.

I considered dedicating a whole chapter to alcohol, but I don't think it is a completely brainless subject. Alcohol is both psychological and sociological. Different alcohols have different alcohol contents. Different alcohols are associated with different settings, socio-economic status and social situations. Different alcohols cost different dollars. Alcohol can be deeply associated with upbringing, religion and morality. Alcohol is also tied to laws that can carry life-altering consequences. Finally, alcohol is a depressant and can easily become addictive.

But so that you are not left without a little brainless wisdom, I offer this. *Do not drink to cope. Do not drink to have fun. Do not drink to release inhibitions. Definitely do not drink to forget. Do not drink because others are drinking. Instead, drink to enjoy the taste of the beverage.* Period. When you order a Coke® or a Sprite® or a Dr.

Pepper®, you are ordering it because you like the taste of it. Apply the same principle to alcohol. That's as brainless as it gets. Let your tummy and your taste buds drive your decision when it comes to alcohol, and then treat it like everything else—with moderation.

Of course, there is a catch. When you start drinking, your ability to make even brainless decisions sometimes goes out the window. Most people typically *keep drinking*, which among other problems adds tons of calories, carbs and sugars. But it gets worse. When we drink, we typically start to crave food, and not the healthy kind. Pretty soon we'll be ordering a pizza or finding a bag of chips or a side of fries. When we drink, we slide toward the unhealthiest of foods.

I didn't believe this until I was drinking at a wedding. Before I knew it, I was scarfing down food from *other people's* plates. I mean I was stuffing it in. It's why there are pizza parlors that are open until 2 a.m. outside of every club in America. People get drunk and they want to eat. Sometimes, they wrongly think that eating will absorb the alcohol and sober them up. It is scientifically unsubstantiated. We just eat simply because alcohol makes us dehydrated and hungry. When we wake up hungover, what do we do? We go out to eat. Sometimes we even start drinking again. It's nuts. Before you know it, you have a vicious cycle and literally thousands of extra calories pouring into your body.

I believe the increased socialization of alcohol has contributed to the diabetes and obesity epidemics in the United States. *Grabbing a drink* is more commonly associated with alcohol than with coffee. Even my most orthodox religious friends indulge in craft beer like it was a harmless hobby. I personally love craft beer and admit that it is my weakness. Add to the exploding craft-beer industry the small batch distillery market. From whisky to vodka to gin and everything in between, cool new products are overshadowing the old brands.

I returned from a business trip to Alaska and went out of my way to bring home a locally distilled bottle of gin. In many ways, I see this as an exciting birth of artistic expression, from labels to bottles to cool names. At the same time, I fear that we forget how *extremely* addictive and damaging that alcohol can be to the mind and body. That's to say nothing about the damage it can do to relationships, employment and families.

My rule of thumb is to treat alcohol like dessert. Enjoy it but don't have it with breakfast, lunch and dinner. That's brainless.

CHAPTER NINE

CONDOMS, SEATBELTS AND HELMETS

USING CONDOMS IS among the most brainless behaviors *and* also the most complex. That's because if you are in the circumstance of needing a condom, then you are balancing your world on the tip of a knife. When condoms enter the conversation, you entertain the possibility of significant life change, including adding another person to the planet. That is the super complex part. The easy part is that they're the best defense against sexually transmitted diseases.

Condoms are cheap and easy to acquire. And while they may be seen as uncool in some social circles, they are the absolute definition of smartness and a sign of maturity and sometimes a source of real sex appeal because it shows you have a brain. You are prepared, and you know the risks.

Google genital herpes on the internet. Little else will scare you like that little image search. That's what you are risking if you have sex without a condom. Syphilis and gonorrhea are equally terrifying searches and far worse diseases. With all our medical advances, no one has found a cure for these STDs. HIV is of course another noteworthy STD that has changed the face of our planet with untold stories of pain and passing.

You've heard all about STDs, but try talking to a man or woman who has genital herpes. When they have a breakout, they might as well wear a chastity belt. They might as well have a lock on their underwear because they won't be dropping their panties for anyone unless it is Halloween and they want to scare you. Sure, there are treatments or prescriptions for a cool $300 per month (or more) to keep those sickening sores from showing up, but even those break-the-bank medications are not sure-fire protectors. They just limit the outbreaks and lessen the severity. Not exactly my definition of money well spent on a risky night of passion.

Of course, that's not to mention oral sores, big nasty sores on your lips for everyone in your family and at your office to see. That's a real nice way to win friends and influence people. Try showing up to the Christmas party with a nice herpes cold sore on your lip. That will make for great watercooler conversation.

Did you get the part about *giving* oozing, nasty sores to your lover or your potential spouse forever? How about giving the gift of cancer? I don't want to go too deep into discussing HPV (human papillomavirus) except to say that according to the Centers for Disease Control and Prevention (CDC), "HPV can cause cervical cancer, plus cancer of the vulva, vagina, penis, or anus. It can also cause cancer in the back of the throat, including the base of the tongue and tonsils." (See: https://www.cdc.gov/std/hpv/stdfact-hpv.htm)

You thought a little oral sex was no big deal? Well, welcome to throat cancer. Not cool. A little unprotected, uninformed sex and you may just transmit cancer. Even worse, it could take a decade to show up. That means that a guy could transmit cancer to a dozen one-night lovers. That's one of the worst parts of HPV. It's got over 100 strains, some of which take care of themselves and disappear, but many that don't. Fortunately, there is a vaccine to prevent HPV for preteens as well as women up to age twenty-six and men twenty-one. That is the best investment and strategic health move you can make. If you are in that age or have kids that age, it is a simple conversation to have with a doctor.

But don't just Google it. That's because, unfortunately, the HPV vaccine conversation got a bit hijacked by some well-intentioned but uninformed advocate groups which thought that getting vaccinated was either an admission of sexual promiscuity or a license to be so. Neither was correct, but once that took hold, it was hard to get the genie back in the bottle. The fact is that boys who are not vaccinated can be carriers and give it to the most chaste, virgin bride one day if she has not been vaccinated. That is what the HPV vaccination shots aim to prevent. Plain and simple. Boys need the vaccine so that they don't spread cancer but also because there is currently no way to test whether boys have the virus.

I hate to get into the vaccination conversation because it is so emotional and divisive, but for goodness' sake, get the facts. Granted, that will cause you to use your brain a little, but I don't see a lot of people rejecting the polio vaccine once they have witnessed someone with polio. Similarly, try talking to the mother who gave her own child a disease because she didn't vaccinate him. Or consider the story of a mother who had never been vaccinated and almost had to tell her own newborn child goodbye after she contracted cancer that could have been prevented.

I'm not here to solve the vaccination debate, but carry a condom and use it. Be brainless. Men *and* women. Tuck one in your pocket or your purse and you will never be unprepared.

But remember, like the ads tell you in micro print, no condom is 100 percent safe, especially when it comes to genital herpes. I have friends who got women pregnant while wearing a condom and others who got STDs wearing them, so act responsibly even while your hormones are telling you otherwise.

The most important thing to protect is your brain and your heart.

Sex, even disease-free sex, is often full of psychological diseases called *regret, guilt, obligation, miscommunication, expectation,* etc. Sex isn't going anywhere. People aren't going to stop having sex or wanting sex, so there is no reason to jump into sex. Period. If you are dying to have sex with someone, then you will be dying to have sex with them tomorrow. And in many cases, the sex you thought you wanted with them in the evening will vanish in the daylight. Sad but true, and you will be forever grateful that you didn't consummate the act.

BRAINLESS SEATBELTS

Seatbelts are the absolute definition of brainless. In fact, when I drive to the end of the driveway without my seatbelt, I feel like a moron. That's because seatbelts have been proven 1,000 times over to keep people alive. Period. It's a fact. You can argue the rightness or wrongness of laws, but you can't argue with the facts.

And they don't just save you from the grave, they save you from a life of prosthetic devices or wheelchairs or worse. In addition to possibly having your limbs amputated or being hooked up to a ventilator for the rest of your life, you just might never drive again. Think about *that* for a second. We all take our daily freedom and self-determination for granted. We jump in our cars and go wherever and whenever we want. That life can end in a millisecond. If the risk of eating the rest of your meals through a straw doesn't motivate you, maybe not being able to drive will.

So, let's agree that you won't be jumping in the car to grab a gallon of milk without buckling up. Got it? No more carpool pickups without buckling in the kids. Got it? No more driving to work, juggling your coffee and phone, without snapping that seatbelt. Got it? If you fail to do this freaking basic, brainless act, then be prepared to live a life of complete dependence on other people. Ask any kid. It sucks.

It's bizarre that we rarely take the time to pause and consider the real-life implications of being disabled. We might remember a high school driver's education video showing people flying through the windshield, but did those videos ever show Johnny *after the wreck*, at the swimming pool in the summer being lifted out of his wheelchair into the pool while the other kids did flips off the diving board? Nope. Few safety videos ever show life after the accident. They should.

Maybe you have been in a car wreck and no one got hurt. Thrilling. Maybe you just smashed your car, and while it was a pain to deal with the mountains of insurance forms and phone calls, no one died. No one bled out on your backseat carpet. That's wonderful. But it's a mixed blessing because you may not have learned your lesson.

Recently, a bartender told me that he just got out of the Marine Corps. He was visiting a buddy who took him for a ride in his new BMW. They were taking corners at 85 MPH, and just as they were headed into the final curve the bartender decided to put on his seatbelt. Within seconds of the seatbelt's metal clicking together, the BMW flew out of control and flipped over three times. This Marine Corps sergeant, who had survived military tours of duty in Libya and Iraq, nearly died on a South Carolina back road. Only his seatbelt saved him.

The reality is that over 1.2 million people die in car crashes every single year according to the World Health Organization. That's a hefty number, but it gets worse. *Fifty million are injured or disabled* every 365 days in car wrecks. Yep. Fifty million. Now think about your family that will be impacted, all because you didn't want to take the time to buckle up. That would be the worst, having your family wipe your butt or feed you every single meal for the rest of your life because you wouldn't take responsibility for strapping yourself into a 2,000-pound hunk of metal called a car.

And if you happen to be reading this and are age thirty or younger, please understand that death-by-car is the number one cause of death for people under age thirty. Please tell people that when you ask them to buckle up in your car. Tell them you aren't a bad driver, but you are about to drive alongside a ton of people who are.

You see, few people ever see the wreck coming. No one *intends* to wreck. Wrecks come out of nowhere. Drivers are blindsided. They are absolutely tapping their foot to the music or reaching for their coffee cup one minute, and the next minute they are catapulted and getting run over by their own car.

A woman recently spoke at an event I attended. She is now in her mid-forties and unable to bare children because of an auto accident that she was involved in at age twelve. She wasn't seriously injured in the wreck—so everyone *thought*. Unfortunately, the impact disrupted her newly developing reproductive parts. No one knew it at the time, and no one even thought to check them out. Can you imagine not being able to enjoy grandchildren simply because you didn't require your own kid to buckle up in the backseat. We certainly can't control much in this world, but wearing a seatbelt is something we can. It's a powerful way to prevent a lot of pain and suffering.

Sure, we've all heard the stories from people who found a news article about someone in Peoria, Illinois, who survived a deadly car crash because she *wasn't* wearing a seatbelt. Sure, that happens, but please don't play those odds. The risk of losing is too big.

Sadly, one of the biggest excuses for not wearing a seatbelt is that people don't want to wrinkle their clothes. Hello? News flash, blood stains are a heck of a lot harder to get out of your clothes than wrinkles. And shards of windshield glass will really do a number on your blouse. Dry cleaners suck at getting plasma out of your favorite suit.

Sure, it messes up my tie. Sure, it is uncomfortable with a bulky overcoat in the middle of winter. Yes, it is hard to fasten the seatbelt with gloves on. But when those stupid thoughts go through my mind, I stop and imagine how hard it will be to navigate my wheelchair on the icy sidewalk with gloves on. I think about how uncomfortable it will be to wait for someone to take my overcoat off *for me* because I can't move my arms.

I pay good money to get every one of my shirts dry cleaned, and while I hate getting them wrinkled, I still buckle up. At least people need to come up with better excuses for being downright dumb.

Ok. Do you get it now? Fastening your seatbelt is the absolute number one brainless act. As we'll discuss, smoking is completely asinine. But it's addictive. Not wearing a condom is asinine. But the heat of the moment can cloud your brain. *Seatbelts, however, have no such limiting factors.*

You might really think that you are invincible, or you simply want to play the odds. Fine, but please think of your passengers. They are not in control of your vehicle. They don't have mirrors in the backseat. They don't have a brake pedal. Please think of them and think about your life if you end up killing one of them. Think about going back to work or to your home after killing a neighbor's kid or your work colleague or your sister. Those scenarios are more horrifying to me than hurting myself. Please promise that you will not drive or ride without a seatbelt. Please commit to making it your brainless behavior forever. And buckle up in your Uber or Lyft. It is easy to get in the backseat of an Uber and feel a false sense of security. Also, many of us rarely ride in the backseat of a car and are therefore unaccustomed to buckling up. We feel that we are protected by the seats in front of us. Nothing could be further from the truth. My friend jumped in an Uber with his fiancée and headed to dinner. In a matter of minutes his Uber was T-boned by a red Ferrari. No joke. What are the chances? A Ferrari slammed into them and sent them to the hospital because they were not wearing seatbelts.

PROTECT YOUR BRAINLESS BRAIN

One memorable Fourth of July, I took my kids to one of the longest bike trails in the nation. I was pumped. It was going to be great. I had mapped it out and planned where we could get off the trail and grab some ice cream. I mounted the bikes onto the car (never an easy task in and of itself). I checked the air pressure in the tires. I filled the water bottles. I psyched up the kids and headed for the trail. We pulled in and I fought for a prime parking spot. I removed the bikes from the car rack without throwing out my back or blowing any blood vessels and we mounted up.

Before we took one full revolution of the crankshaft, a bike-mounted cop rode over and told me that everyone needed to have a helmet. I was stunned. We were going to ride on a flat paved path that was straight as an arrow. It was the baby trail of all trails. I wore a bike helmet when I went hurtling down mountain bike trails, wiping out at every turn, but this was totally different.

Apparently, helmets are the law in my state, and no one told me. The cop sent us packing. I remounted the bikes on the car, reinserted the children and headed to Walmart to buy four helmets. We dropped $100 and headed back to the trail. As we arrived, it started pouring rain.

One thing I can't stand to see are parents who outfit their kids with bike helmets only to troll behind their kids without wearing a helmet themselves. Not only does it confuse the kids and communicate that adults don't have to protect themselves, but it puts the parents at massive risk. They need to ask themselves, *Who will care for my kids after I get a traumatic brain injury?*

Nearly 1,000 people die every year in bike wrecks, according to federal statistics. I won't go into the state-by-state death stats because the only thing you need to think about is your brains or the brains of your loved ones splayed out on the pavement.

Unlike cars, motorcycles and bicycles and scooters have zero around you to protect you. There are no seatbelts on bikes. There are no airbags on bikes. There is nothing between you and the pavement or between you and the steel panels of a speeding car slamming into you.

Don't even get me started on scooters. They popped up like weeds everywhere, and I have yet to see a single person riding one of them with a helmet. As I write this, there are countless lawsuits against scooter manufacturers due to traumatic brain injuries, comas, paralysis and surgeries all resulting from scooter accidents. They should come with a helmet attached to them, but since they don't, you need to throw a helmet in your backpack or clip one onto your briefcase if you intend to go for a ride. Sure, it's bulky. Sure, it's a pain. Sure, it looks goofy. I get it, but you must change your perspective. Troll around your helmet as a badge of honor. Understand that it is a message to the world that you are educated. You are intelligent. Tell the world that you want to be the one visiting the hospital patient who crashed, not the one being visited. It's as simple as that. Do it or don't ride.

A safer option is to simply walk. Walking will always be 10,000 times better for your health than even the safest scooter on the planet.

I was knocked off my bike by a car one day and my bike was destroyed. It was like a pipe cleaner, all curled and bent up. My legs were seriously scraped up with chunks of pavement embedded in them, but fortunately, my sweet little noggin was perfectly protected by my helmet.

Believe me, I don't think any bike helmet will ever win a fashion award. They certainly give new meaning to *hat hair,* but as I discussed before with regard to seatbelts and dry cleaning, if you are worried about how your hair will look from wearing a helmet, think about your new style after they've shaved half of your skull to perform cranial surgery.

A friend of mine had a brain tumor removed and they used a real technical surgical tool called a *saw.* Yep. They used a power saw on her skull. It's so flipping nasty I could hardly look at the pictures of the ten-inch scar. Sadly, she is now a wig expert. Think about that the next time you consider how a helmet might mess up your hair.

Together, seatbelts, helmets and condoms are super simple, low-cost (or no-cost) decisions that will save your life and that of others. If you can't afford condoms, call up your local health department and they will give you truckloads for free.

TONAL DISCLAIMER

Recently I gave a presentation about prevention. A man I respect told me that I needed to lighten up my message. I needed to make it a little bit warmer. He said that prevention is a hard thing to sell because no one likes to think that bad things will happen to them. He told me that people don't like to think about being impaled by a tree or a fence as a result of a bike or scooter or auto accident. Basically, he was saying that people would prefer to talk about orgasms instead of herpes. No joke. I couldn't agree more. I don't like to think of those things either. But I'm also a father, and part of my job as someone who feels a deep responsibility to my children (and all children) is to think about protecting them as much as possible. As I've said before, we can't prevent everything bad from happening, but I live in a constant state of amazement over how many travesties could have been prevented if someone had taken some utterly simple steps to avoid them. I always tell my kids that newspapers are not filled with normal stories of death and dying. They are filled with stories that are stranger than fiction. Most could have been prevented if people knew the risks associated with certain behaviors and had the guts to lead by example.

Predictably, I won't be *warming up* my approach to prevention. I am going to beat this drum right into your brain. I'm going to tell you what no one else seems to want to tell you. Life is super precious, and we all need to treat it like the priceless treasure it is. There is absolutely nothing more valuable, so we must not be so cavalier.

I hope you don't warm up your own *prevention message* to your friends and family either. Tell them the truth. Tell them the whole story. Tell them that you are not asking them to get their PhD in injury prevention but rather you are sharing the brainless things in this book to help them greatly reduce their chances of watching life go by from a hospital window.

FINAL THOUGHTS

There is strange commonality between helmets, seatbelts and condoms (not to mention life jackets.) What I find fascinating is that our relationship to seatbelts, lifejackets, helmets and condoms is one largely related to vanity. This blows my mind. We would rather be dead than not look cool on the road, on the lake or in the bed. It's time we get over our ridiculous vanity and focus on staying alive so that we can keep combing our own hair, pressing our own shirts and slipping under our own sheets.

CHAPTER TEN

IN YOUR HANDS

THIS CHAPTER IS not about getting a flu shot, but as I write this, over 30,000 people have already died from the flu *this year*, and that's a pretty good motivator to get the shot. I always enjoy watching the news during flu season because they always have a health expert or government official being interviewed. You know what they say? "Wash your hands." Oh, my goodness. Really? That's the expert recommendation? Still? What century are we in? How long have we had running water in the United States? Two hundred years ago, when you had to boil water and pour it in a bowl and then use some kind of expensive powder called soap to wash your hands, it was definitely a challenge. But hello? Today every single restaurant, airport, school, store and office building lets you wash your hands 100 times a day if you want—absolutely free. Of course, in your own home, you pay for the soap and water, but hopefully those two things aren't breaking your monthly budget.

I just can't get over the fact that our most erudite experts and officials must remind people of this brainless act of health. I consider it to be one of the easier tasks in my day, but somehow people just won't do it. I'm stumped as to an explanation for this phenomenon. Maybe they don't like water on their hands. Maybe they are afraid they will splash on their clothes. Maybe they think it will just take way too much of their valuable time. Maybe, like the proverbial phrase attests, "they think their shit don't stink." They literally think that they are somehow different and better than the rest of us pathetic slobs who have to wash germs from our hands.

If you pay attention, you will still find some signs in public bathrooms that show step-by-step instructions, with a diagram, of how to wash your hands. It is mind blowing. Whenever I teach about health communication, I use those signs as a joke, because I really can't accept the idea that people need a tutorial on how to apply soap to their hands, turn them over and over under a stream of water and then dry them. It depresses me. Maybe in emerging countries that don't have running water, but not in the modern world.

People who don't wash their hands not only risk harming themselves, but they spread the risk, too. The sign in the bathroom should read, *If you don't wash your hands, please do not leave the bathroom.* And certainly do not touch the table in the restaurant, or the breadbasket or the pen to sign your bill, or the elevator button or the escalator railing, or shake *my* hand!

You may be one of the fooled masses that thinks washing your hands is overrated. You have read articles that say that too much hand washing prevents your body from building up a strong immune system. I don't like being the one to tell you, but too much hand washing is simply not a risk. I wish it was. I wish it was a national crisis instead of communicable diseases. For goodness sakes, there are apps and devices that remind doctors to wash their hands and even track their handwashing. If anyone doesn't need reminding, I figured it was the doctors who are around germs all day, but apparently, they need reminding too.

So, if that's your concern, you are thinking way too much. Just do what your mother told you to do and wash up.

Let's review. Men touch their penises daily when going to the bathroom or dressing or other more intimate activities. In doing so, they are placing their hands on that naturally sweaty part of their body. Those same men then shake hands with other people and before long we get a nice cross-pollination of penile germs. Then we hit the elevator button and leave them there for the next unsuspecting soul. On and on it goes. The copier machine, the refrigerator door, the doorknob, the everything. Our world is one big petri dish of bacteria, viruses and fungal germs.

There is the false presumption that men are the real hand-washing offenders and women always clean up after themselves, but that isn't supported by the evidence that is collected from public bathroom doorknobs and stalls. Women can theoretically get away with hands-free urination, but it's the teaming array of germs that live in the bathroom that are still at large. Then, just like men, women emerge from the bathroom and begin touching the same array of light switches and buttons and surfaces to spread their germs to the rest of the world.

I don't know what goes on in women's bathrooms, but I am always amazed at how many men I see exiting the bathroom stalls and urinals and walk right out the door without even glancing at the sink. It is like it doesn't exist or it is a place only for the weak. Perhaps it seems unmanly to wash. I wish I could stand at the bathroom door and put a sticker on everyone's back who leaves without washing that reads, *I didn't wash my hands after I took a dump.* I would love to see people's reactions. (Will someone please do that sociological study and let me know the results?)

COVER YOUR MOUTH

I know I've just been talking about bathroom germs. Those are the tip of the germ iceberg. The real dangers are being coughed and sneezed out of our body and into the air, across our computer keyboards, the lunch counter, the remote control, the credit card reader, the car steering wheel, the airplane seat, etc. All of us cough and sneeze our germs into the path of others. Therefore, our parents raise us to cover our mouth when we sneeze or cough. Polite training of course, but not exactly healthy. If we use our hands, then we turn around and shake someone's else's hand or touch something, the game goes on. During flu season, we think a lot about limiting the people we hug or kiss, but we need to be aware that people all around us are sick every single day of the year, not just during flu season.

People routinely come to the office, go shopping or go somewhere out in public while carrying a seemingly inconsequential cold. They might say, "I just have the sniffles," or "I must have allergies." But it's very possible that those sniffles include a virus or serious respiratory infection. Kids are germ factories who aren't exactly the best hand-washing practitioners. They touch everything, often shoving their hands in their mouth. They then hold their parents' hands.

The goal is not to avoid coughing or sneezing but rather to clean one's hands often, and always before touching the things that we put into our mouth, such as food. Washing your hands before eating is totally brainless, and washing them after needs to become as automatic since we often will lick our fingers or pick food from our teeth while eating.

We often tell children to wash their hands *after* a meal to get the ketchup or greasy French fry oil off them, but in fact we are helping them remove their own saliva as well, since most kids end up with their fingers in their mouth at some point in the meal. Same with adults. Just picture someone eating buffalo wings. Unlike children, however, adults typically know how to use a napkin and so they simply wipe or dry their hands after they eat, removing all outward signs of germs. But wiping is not the same as washing.

I love sitting in frequent-flyer clubs at the airport and watching businesspeople drink cocktails and snarf up Chex mix, nuts and other finger foods. I watch them lick their fingers and pick peanuts from their teeth. Then, suddenly, a business associate walks up from another flight and they jump up and extend their hand. *Lovely.*

Try going to the gym and touching the sweaty knobs and buttons and bars and then wiping everyone's germs across your dripping brow with your own unwashed hands. Then of course you pass along the favor by spreading your slop onto the bars and buttons for others to share. As I've said, I love the gym, but I'm a big utilizer of sanitizer and I encourage you to follow suit.

Washing our hands isn't just a nice thing to do that keeps us from spreading germs and disease to our fellow man. It is necessary because we take our dirty digits and wipe them, shove them and touch them all over our bodies. We pick our noses with dirty fingers, then we rub our eyes. Some of us like to pick our teeth, inserting our fingers halfway down our throat. We love to itch the inside of our ears, pretending that our finger is a Q-Tip®, and then share the contents. *All the while, we wonder why we are sick.* For goodness' sake, our eyes, mouths and noses and ears are all orifices that have permeable membranes, which means that germs can be easily transferred into the bloodstream. That's why many medicines are given though the eyes or ears or nose. These entry points to the body absorb germs as readily as they absorb medicine and do so incredibly quickly with few barriers.

I'm not Martha Stewart or Emily Post. I'm not interested in etiquette. I'm interested in preventing nauseating sickness. Keeping you healthy and keeping you alive. Here's one easy way to accomplish that: Use hand sanitizer when you can't wash. Please don't buy into the insanity that too much sanitizer doesn't allow you to build up a strong immune system. Maybe that would be true if you bathed in it, but believe me, there are enough bugs and germs landing on the rest of your body and flying up your nose and into your ears and eyes to keep your immune system working overtime. Keep a bottle of sanitizer in your car or throw one in your office drawer, briefcase, purse or gym bag. Just have it available for a squirt when you leave the gym or the gas station or the port-o-potty. You get the idea.

According to many studies, the fingernails are the dirtiest parts of our bodies. Dirt easily collects under them and stays there. Then we pop a zit or scratch our nose or pick our teeth with these dirty tools. Therefore, washing your hands *well*, so well as to dislodge some of that dirt under your nails, is the ultimate gold standard.

I was recently washing my hands in a public restroom when a guy walked in. He immediately started washing his hands, and only after thoroughly doing so did he walk to the urinal. I was amazed. I had heard about this genius move but rarely ever witnessed it out in the wild. Sure enough, this evolved human decided that after touching the doors and chairs and elevator buttons and subway poles, he would rather clean up before transferring all of that filth to his own body.

So, try this new idea: wash, pee and wash again. *WPW.* Your hands won't come off. I promise.

Practice the Golden Rule. Even if you don't think you have germs like everyone else, just go ahead and wash your hands because you would appreciate it if others would wash theirs. Lead by example. It's as simple as that and we'll all be glad you did.

AVOID HOSPITALS

A few final words on germ exposure. Hospitals are healing places, but they're also cauldrons of germs. If you must go to the hospital, get in and out of the hospital as fast as humanly possible.

According to the CDC, healthcare-associated infections (HAIs) affect 5 to 10 percent of hospitalized patients in the US every year. That translates to approximately 1.7 million HAIs in US hospitals annually, resulting in *99,000 deaths* and rack up an estimated $20 billion in healthcare costs. Almost 100,000 people perish in the hospital due to things they contract in the hospital. Got it?

Healthcare-associated infections are infections people get while they are receiving health care for *another* condition. HAIs can occur at any healthcare facility, including hospitals, ambulatory surgical centers, end-stage renal disease facilities, and long-term care facilities. HAIs can be caused by bacteria, fungi, viruses, or other, less common pathogens.

Stay out needs to be your main mantra, and *get out* needs to follow it up. It doesn't make any difference how fancy or big or expensive your hospital is, you will always be at risk when you put a bunch of sick people in a closed building. Think about that. It's a no-brainer. Plus, if you are presumably sick when you go in there, your immune system is likely already compromised.

I respect hospitals and the people who work saving lives. They are high-tech hubs but still can't purify or safeguard their environment enough to prevent a bunch of deaths by infection, complication or negligence. We are all human, and even the best of the best cannot completely prevent human error, oversight, germs or dirty air particles. Like I said, this is a multi-faceted, complex topic with solutions that are far from brainless. But staying out of them is.

There are some factors that raise the risk of HAIs, such as injections, surgery, catheters, improper use of antibiotics and diseases transferred between patients and healthcare workers. But what are you going to do? If you are going in, you don't really have a lot of choices or control. The only real defense is your body's condition *prior* to going into the hospital. It has been well documented that your ability to handle HAIs and medical procedures of any kind depends on the strength of your immune system and your overall historical health. If you are typically a healthy individual, you will resist disease better and bounce back faster.

Lastly, when you do find yourself in the hospital, drink tons of water, only take the pain pills if you absolutely have to, wash your hands constantly (especially if you shake hands with the doctor) and get the heck out of there as soon as possible.

CHAPTER ELEVEN

THE WORST HABIT

OK, BUCKLE UP for this chapter. It's probably going to get offensive. It might just be the harshest chapter in the book if you smoke or know someone who smokes. Don't judge me because I'm not judging anyone. I'm just the messenger and I'm going to say it like it is.

Most things in this book are not new to you, and certainly the ill effects of smoking is hardly breaking news. If you don't smoke, fabulous. You have already saved yourself from literally hundreds of maladies, including increased risk for hundreds more, such as diabetes, cancer, heart disease, high blood pressure and stroke. You are one of the truly smart people on planet Earth.

That's because smoking is just plain stupid. You hear that it's dangerous and damaging, but no one tells you that it is moronic. But even that is a major understatement. Why not just call a spade a spade? People call it an expensive habit, addictive and hard to quit, but the only message that we need to promote is how completely idiotic it is.

Until every human recognizes that smoking is a sign of monumental ignorance, then people will continue this dirty, disgusting, deadly behavior that hurts everyone else on the planet.

Nothing tops it as a baseless, pointless activity. There is absolutely no redeeming quality that comes from smoking.

I'm not saying that there aren't *reasons* that people smoke, they are just bad reasons. And of course, it is brutally hard to quit. I get it. But it's hard to quit any addiction like porn, gambling or drugs. How about alcoholics, for goodness sakes? When did we give them a pass? When did we tell them to keep drinking, but simply take their flask onto the drinking patio or the designated drinking deck at the airport, the way we provide special places for people to smoke?

The double standard is truly audacious. The English language doesn't have enough words to describe the utter mental depravity of someone who smokes in the twenty-first century given the massive knowledge and messaging we have on the subject.

Of course, there are other tobacco products, but everyone focuses on cigarettes because it is the lion's share of the problem, but cigars, e-cigs, vapes and hookahs are equally stupid. Hell, why limit what we smoke? Why not wrap up some dog feces in a paper towel and smoke that? It wouldn't be half as bad for you. Dog feces doesn't contain over 4,000 chemicals that are in cigarettes. I promised that I wouldn't force you to use your brain too much in this book, but just remember the number *43*. That's the number of actual, proven, cancer-causing compounds that are in a single cigarette. I could bore you with all the science about what smoking does to your blood vessels, heart valves and nerves, but all you really need to know is that it gives you wrinkly skin, ugly teeth, nasty breath and erectile dysfunction. Even smokers report not liking the smell of their clothes or their breath.

Believe me, I understand addiction. It is powerful beyond words. The average smoker tries to quit nine times before the addictive hooks in their brains are finally, painfully ripped out. If you are reading this book, then hopefully you care about your health and hopefully don't smoke. But you also likely know someone who does smoke, and that is the real focus of my rant. We must work together to create a smoke-free world. Why? Because secondhand smoke is as insidious as firsthand smoke. It doesn't just make your clothes smell, it kills people. It kills kids and pets. The CDC featured a man in one of its anti-smoking campaigns who was killed by secondhand smoke in the casino where he worked. He never smoked a cigarette in his life. That's not fair. Why should people be killed because someone else doesn't care about killing themselves?

The anti-smoking efforts have been expansive and intense. The federal government began by requiring warning labels on ads and cigarette packages. Then it banned most advertising. Then it sued the tobacco industry. Once that multi-year, multi-billion-dollar litigation was over, they legislated the smokers out on the sidewalk with the Smokefree Air Laws. From office buildings to restaurants to parks, the smokers were told to get out. Literally. Then they socked it to their wallets though exorbitant cigarette taxes. Just recently one city raised the cost of a pack of cigs to thirteen dollars. Lastly, they focused on secondhand smoke, and people began to demand that their neighbor put out their cigarette before walking across the street. Only after they learned that someone else's actions could harm them and their children did non-smokers begin to turn on smokers.

My point is that society approached it from all angles, financial and legislative and social, but not until the regular people started ostracizing smokers did the anti-smoking crusade really gain traction. That is what must continue to happen with smoking and overeating and failure to exercise. I dream of a day when someone stops ordering fettuccini alfredo that overflows the plate or stops bragging about how they sat on the couch all day because of positive peer pressure, or better yet, *positive health pressure.*

Of course, I am not talking about shaming. I'm talking about *compassionate intolerance.* That simply means that we love the smoker but will not sit by and tolerate their decision to indulge in life-killing behavior. We need to grow an intolerance to all kinds of unhealthy mental and physical and emotional behaviors, because ultimately, it harms those we love either directly or indirectly.

It harms our community, our nation and our society. We must recognize the need for tough love when it comes to health. It really is a matter of life and death.

And for all those people who know someone who lived to the age of 100 and who smoked a pack a day, I say, "So what?" That's like saying I know someone who jumped out of an airplane without a parachute and lived. Fabulous. Most don't survive or don't survive *well*. And these killers are costly. Chronic obstructive pulmonary disease (COPD) is the third most common cause of death in the US and costs over $50 billion every single year, according to the National Center for Biotechnology Information. Imagine footing your part of that bill. News flash, you do. You pay for it. Every year in taxes. And what about emphysema? What about ER trips and hospital stays related to that? Smokers can say goodbye to the retirement beach house and hello to monthly medical bills. Seriously, say hello to weekly dialysis appointments or shopping for glucose meters, because if smoking doesn't kill you, something else will, like heart disease or diabetes.

Hey, I get it. In the past, even I wanted to be the Marlboro Man. Sadly Marlboro had to get multiple actors to play in their ads because many of them died from smoking related diseases. What tragic irony.

I was recently visiting Greece, and every time I would mention that I worked in public health or mentioned my amazement at how many Greeks smoke, they would laugh (yes laugh!) and tell me that a Greek breakfast consisted of coffee and a cigarette. That's funny to them but insane to me. Especially considering that Greece is in an economic morass.

Cigarette smoking is linked to economic loss according to every scholarly paper every written. The workforce ends up missing work due to illness, health insurance costs skyrocket, the healthcare system is stretched, accidents happen, fires happen, trash accumulates. People are destroying their lives, their communities and their economies that are responsible for providing them with a job, health insurance, education and safety, all of which are suffering in countries with high rates of smoking. It's insanity. There is not one redeeming aspect to smoking. Not even at the Greek breakfast table.

Crazier still is the fact that all over Europe, you will find printed on cigarette cartons stomach-churning pictures of people spitting up blood. They have actual photos of gaping holes in the human throat and naked men curled up in the fetal position with the words, *Cigarette smoking leads to erectile dysfunction.* That's certainly not widely known or discussed, and frankly that would do it for me. Once I learned that the Marlboro Man couldn't get it up, the macho illusion would be completely over. Cold turkey.

The reality of a national obsession with smoking is of course not limited to Greece. According to the World Health Organization, 25 percent of all economic costs associated with smoking come from Russia, Brazil, China and India. Those countries already have a million problems to manage, without having the economic killer of smoking layered on top.

SIMPLY STOP

Sadly, the path to ending the insanity begins with terminology. The healthcare and public health community preach the word *cessation*, which simply means "the fact or process of ending or being brought to an end." I prefer the word *stop*. Everyone knows that word, no matter language or literacy level. It is not ambiguous in any way. *Stop* is both the goal *and* the process. Second, everyone and their mother has a cessation program, from private companies to nonprofits to the government. One of the hardest parts of quitting must be choosing which program to follow. Add to that, dozens of companies have products on the market to stop the cravings, manage the withdrawals or replace the activities related to smoking. My highly sophisticated Google research revealed *twenty* different flavors or formats of Nicorette® gum alone. According to Grand View Research, the global cessation and nicotine de-addiction market is $20 billion annually. (See: https://www.grandviewresearch.com/press-release/global-smoking-cessation-nicotine-de-addiction-market)

While I am a big fan of business, I'd love to put smoking cessation companies out of business because everyone just stopped smoking. They put down their cigarettes and picked up a pack of gum, a cup of coffee, an energy drink, a knitting needle, a jump rope or a gym membership. They started blowing up the 1-800-QUITNOW support line and started asking their friends to hold them accountable. They simply stopped. Of course, it will be hell on earth for a period of time, but according to WebMD, the body's self-healing process starts *right away*. They chronicle the process by the minute and by the hour below:

20 minutes: "In less time than it takes to watch a sitcom, your body's already getting better. After 20 minutes, your pulse and blood pressure start to drop back to normal. And your hands and feet warm up to their usual temperature."

8 hours: "By the end of a work day, you have half the amount of nicotine and carbon monoxide in your blood. Why does that matter? Carbon monoxide is a chemical in cigarettes, and it crowds out oxygen in your blood. That causes problems from your muscles to your brain because they don't get the oxygen they need. But as the chemical's levels drop, your oxygen gets back to normal. On the flip side, it's likely you already feel some early cravings and doubts. That's normal. But they usually last just 5-10 minutes. To get you through, try to find ways to distract yourself until the feeling passes. You could try making a craving playlist, chewing gum, or sipping water."

12 hours: "Halfway through your first day, your carbon monoxide level is back to normal. And your heart will thank you. Now it doesn't have to pump so hard to try to get enough oxygen to your body."

24 hours: "If you smoke a pack a day, you're twice as likely to have a heart attack as a nonsmoker. But go one full day without a cigarette, and you've already lowered your chances. That's huge."

The CDC reports, "Within two to five years after quitting smoking, your risk for stroke may reduce to about that of a nonsmoker's. If you quit smoking, your risks for cancers of the mouth, throat, esophagus, and bladder drop by half within five years. Ten years after you quit smoking, your risk for dying from lung cancer drops by half."

Ten years from now might just put you right on time for your daughter's wedding or your son's graduation or your thirtieth wedding anniversary or your long-awaited retirement. Regardless, your overall risk for a life-ending stroke or heart attack starts to go down the very day you trash your smokes, the very same day that you decide that enough is enough. The very same day you stop, you begin to win.

If you are a smoker who wants to quit, I salute you. I know many people who have successfully quit, and it remains one of their greatest life accomplishments. That's because it is like climbing Mt. Everest. It is incredibly hard, but incredibly doable.

The hardest things in life are the best. Hardness creates diamonds. Hardness is nothing compared to life on a ventilator. *That's* hard. There is a great community of sojourners on the same trek to termination. The rewards are beyond words. The results are beyond your imagination. Your loved ones will not love you more, but they will be able to love you longer, simply because you will be around longer for them to love. I give you permission to put down this book right now and pick up your phone to dial 1-800-QUITNOW. Just do it.

Ultimately, we can't control how long any of us will live, but we can greatly influence the quality of those years and reducing the risk that we will be hooked up to cords and cables for years upon end. Smoking, on the other hand, nearly guarantees that suffering will punctuate a grotesque, miserable end to life. So please take a deep drag on your last cigarette and then screw your head on tightly and stop with the excuses. Stop putting your loved ones at risk. Stop putting your friends, employer and community at risk. Stop putting your pets at risk. Deal with the withdrawal and embrace a new reality. Even the worst withdrawals will be better than coughing up blood. It's brainless.

ABOUT KIDS

Just a note about youth smoking. It is a complex, psycho-social dynamic that deserves an entirely separate book. Moreover, youth smoking has different physiological effects on developing brain tissue, and organs. I hate youth smoking more than just about anything. It is the fastest path to cancer and it often leads to alcohol and drug abuse. Additionally, it hurts your studies and your career as well as your wallet and your relationships. If your kids smoke, check out the TruthInitiative.org or other youth-focused, anti-smoking organizations. They have great resources and you will help them avoid an avalanche of pain.

If you are a teen smoker, then please understand that smoking is the furthest thing from being cool in the world. It is an advertisement that you are a follower, you lack self-confidence, you have zero ambition, and you are clueless that people don't want to hire you, date you or pay for your disgusting, deadly habit. If your friends smoke, either find new friends or help them to find truly cool ways to stand out, be accepted, and succeed in life without a cigarette hanging from their lips. Otherwise, please recognize that the world is against you and you will suffer in a thousand ways. Hot Instagram models with cigarettes between their fingers are the best advertisements for failure. They are a red flag for employers and a detour sign for daters. There are many more ways to look cool, win friends and succeed in life—starting with your personality.

CHAPTER TWELVE

DARK SUNSHINE

ROCKY SAID IT BEST. "Life aint all sunshine and rainbows." That's especially true when the sunshine gives you cancer. Unprotected overexposure to the sun is not the only way that you can get skin cancer, but it's the leading cause. Fortunately, it's easily addressable. Please read on.

Now, don't worry. I'm not telling you to avoid laying out and getting a tan. Nor am I going to tell you to wear a hat 24/7 or long sleeves in the summer (like my dermatologist tells me). Those are very good ideas, but they often require using your brain to plan, and that's not the focus of this book. We need *brainless* solutions. You should pay attention to the weather forecast, pack the hat (and the hairbrush after removing the hat), wear the long sleeves, pack the sunscreen in your briefcase or backpack, etc. It can be tricky.

What isn't hard is to remember is to wear *sunscreen* at the pool or beach. It's a simple as carrying it with you. A lot of other people are using it. They are spraying it and smearing it. It's on display all around you. Plus, you are usually wearing your swimsuit and you grab a towel (and maybe a book or headphones), and you are out the door. It's not that hard to toss sunscreen into your beach bag as well. Fortunately, to help us remember, the sunscreen manufacturers have done a killer job of ingraining in our heads that we need sunscreen if we want to look good. Hey, I said earlier that I don't care how we get to health as long as we get there. If they want to appeal to our vanity, that's fine with me.

I love the sun and I love the way I look with a tan. Therefore, I indulge in the sun, but not without sunscreen that I apply early and often. That's the key. It's common to see people lather up when they first arrive to their lounge chair and then forget about it. They sweat, and the sunscreen drips off them. Worse, they jump in the pool or ocean and off it comes. Even the sweat-resistant sport brands of sunscreen dissipate from exposure to wetness.

According to Dr. Arthur Perry, a board-certified plastic surgeon, and an adjunct associate professor at Columbia University, "sunscreens need to be rubbed into the skin twenty minutes *before* sun exposure. They do a pretty good job at blocking UV light, but they actually get used up as the sun shines on them. In fact, some sunscreens lose as much as 90 percent of their effectiveness in just one hour, so they need to be reapplied often."

That twenty-minute sunscreen *warm up* was news to me. I admit, my mom never told me that. Unfortunately, it is kind of tricky given that I usually have clothes on twenty minutes before I hit the beach, even if it is just a T-shirt and shorts. Plus, I'm not a huge fan of lubing up and then putting on my clothes, but if you can handle those little hurdles, your skin will thank you for it. If you can't, then just get the stuff on your skin as soon as you disrobe.

At the risk of getting way too technical for our purposes, I want to share a little known but highly logical (*brainless*) fact about most sunscreens. Most of your typical lotions and spray sunscreens are made up of chemicals that must be absorbed into the skin to be effective. The chemicals then absorb the harmful UV radiation and release heat. That makes complete sense. However, what is also unfortunate about that is that anything that gets absorbed into our skin passes *into* our body. The potential problem is that absorbed chemicals make their way into our bloodstream and into our organs, which has people questioning the impact of that. You can learn more at this website, among other places. (See: https://www.livescience.com/32666-how-does-sunscreen-work.html)

Research has raised concerns that *some chemicals* in sunscreen can cause cancer. According to a report by the Environmental Working Group (EWG), scientists found that oxybenzone absorbs into the skin and is present in urine long after sunscreen is applied. Therefore, the EWG recommends not using those sunscreens on children. I'm not a rocket scientist, but it seems to me that if it is not good for kids, it probably isn't all that good for adults either. While it might not hurt me, I won't be stocking up on it.

Fortunately, there are *two inorganic-chemical kinds of sunscreen* that block the sun's rays (UVA and UVB) just like paint blocks sun from your house. Those sunscreens contain zinc oxide and titanium oxide. Even better, the famous *white lifeguard nose* from using zinc oxide sunscreen in the 1950s is a thing of the past. Today's manufacturers make *clear zinc* and titanium products, so you can be extra safe and not look weird.

According to LiveScience.com writer Kristina Grifantini, most organizations recommend using sunscreen with an SPF between 15 and 50 (SPF ratings higher than 50 have not been proven to be more effective than SPF 50). A sunscreen with an SPF of 15 protects against about 93 percent of UVB rays, and one with an SPF of 30 protects against 97 percent of rays, according to the Mayo Clinic. No SPF can block 100 percent of UV rays.

Because most people do not use enough sunscreen and because sunscreen tends to rub or wash off, the Skin Cancer Foundation recommends reapplying sunscreen within two hours *regardless of its SPF strength* and using at least an ounce (a shot-glassful) for maximum protection. A shot glass of lotion is a large amount, but it is easy to rub into the skin in short order. Trickier are spray sunscreens. You'd have to be spraying a long time to fill up a shot glass. Worse is that if there is a breeze blowing, then a ton of your protection is gone with the wind before it hits your skin.

While hunting for long chemical names on sunscreen bottles is not exactly brainless, it might be worth your time. I don't want to recommend a brand or a kind of sunscreen because as soon as I do some new study will reveal that it gives you tumors. If you want to research the world of super safe sunscreens, then Google will be happy to help you. Just be wary of those on the internet who say things like using peanut butter is the best sunscreen. Keep your body butters for the bedroom, not the beach.

In the meantime, to be completely brainless, please slather on at least some kind of sunscreen every couple of hours when you're tanning or walking or playing sports. *It's like wearing your underwear. Don't forget to put it on and don't forget to change it.*

I like a tan face, but I don't want one that is burnt, blotchy, peeling or with wrinkles. If you are only going to protect one place on your body, protect your head and face. After all that's where your eyes, ears, nose, mouth and brain live. Keep those guys especially healthy. Plus, your face is the last place you want the surgeon to remove a hockey-puck-sized melanoma.

A few years ago, I started using self-bronzing sunscreen. It protects me from the sun while attempting to make my skin the color I want to achieve with a tan. Why not kill two birds with one stone? It just makes sense. Of course, some of those products turn your skin orange, so beware of that, and almost all will tan the palms of your hands while applying the lotion, so be sure to wash your hands right afterward. No need to scare your friends and family with tan palms.

But the most brainless behavior of all is the good-ol' hat and sunglasses. They are low cost, they don't wear off, they never cause cancer, and they work every time.

Vitamin D is a hot topic, and if you search you will most certainly find lots of articles on the health benefits of the sun. I would be remiss if I didn't mention how important it is to get a moderate amount of sunlight every day if possible—while protecting your skin.

Due to various reasons, an increasing number of people have become deficient in vitamin D, which can lead to depression, bone and back pain, fatigue, hair loss and muscle pain. One of the easiest ways to get enough vitamin D is from sunlight. Your body makes vitamin D from cholesterol in your body, when your skin is exposed to sunlight. However, it is estimated that 41.6 percent of US adults are deficient in vitamin D. Getting twenty minutes of sunlight a day can be enough to produce all the vitamin D your body needs.

Just ask yourself how you feel on a sunny day versus a rainy day. It's a pretty easy verdict. When we feel better about the day, our bodies feel better too. It's brainless. So, sit outside for a few minutes every day when the sun is shining on a patio. And yes, wear a hat, put sunscreen on your nose, cover your extremities when possible. Don't get burned. Feel happy.

Never forget, getting a sunburn is not a sign of smartness. It is like burning your food in the kitchen. It kills things. It kills cells and it can cause them to mutate. Having just five sunburns or more doubles your chances of getting melanoma, and more people are diagnosed with skin cancer every year than all other cancers combined. Do you need to read that again? Please do. Then tell everyone you know.

TANNING BEDS

I screwed up. Long ago, someone told me that I should use a tanning bed before I went on my first cruise so that I wouldn't burn when I was sailing the high seas. I followed that ill advice and now admit I was a complete idiot not to research tanning beds.

Tanning beds are never the solution to any problem or a safe way to get bronzed. There are tons of studies that explain how tan or pigment-impacted skin reacts when exposed repeatedly to the sun. While the debate rages, the bottom line is that increased sun exposure over time leads to an increased risk for skin cancer. Period. It's logical. It's brainless. Expose anything to more and more light and heat over time and it's going to take its toll. It might dry it out like grilled chicken or change color like cooked pork. Nothing is a guarantee, but it will change in some way, 100 percent of the time.

I don't care if it is a teenager by the pool or an executive who spends every day on the golf course and wears his bronzed skin like a scorecard on his face. A little color is fine. A sun-kissed nose is sweet, or a nice bikini line can be sexy, but more than that is downright idiotic. It is a cultural declaration that your head is in the sand. While most people don't know that 9,500 people get diagnosed with skin cancer *every day*, and *two die from it every hour*, according to the Skin Cancer Foundation, everyone *should know* that too much sun is a bad thing. And when it comes to increasing your risk, tanning beds are the granddaddy. Consider it sickness on steroids.

If you need to get cancer quick, then just turn on the tanning bed bulbs. By the way, tanning beds are the evil friend of Caucasian teenagers everywhere. According to American Academy of Dermatology, nearly 70 percent of tanning salon patrons are Caucasian girls, and melanoma is the second most common cancer in females ages fifteen to twenty-nine. Imagine all of the different cancers that a girl can get, such as breast, cervical or ovarian cancer, along with every other kind common to men *and* women, such as thyroid, bladder, pancreatic and kidney. *Yet melanoma is number two.* It's totally insane.

In 2009, the World Health Organization's International Agency for Research on Cancer classified UV tanning beds as Class 1 human carcinogens. Class 1 is the highest risk category. *Class 1 human carcinogen.* Hello? Do not let your son or daughter tan in those human toasters. Cancel your membership if you have one. Stop lighting the firecracker! This is brainless.

In addition to the common skin cancers, consider a nice case of eye cancer. How about a depressed immune system? How about cataracts and other eye diseases? How about lip cancer and mouth cancer? Mind blowing. All accelerated and accentuated by tanning beds. Just think about the crazy-looking eye goggles they give you in a tanning salon. If you need hyper-intensive sunglasses just to squeeze into a reflective glass coffin, I'm guessing that your unprotected skin is screaming for its life.

Although indoor tanning devices operate on a timer, the exposure to UV rays can vary based on the age and type of light bulbs, according to the CDC. Worse yet, in 2014 a study showed that the newer tanning beds are *no safer* than the older ones. Disappointing, because that is the line that every bronzed model working at the tanning salon will tell you. By the way, I'm not a fan of anyone working at a tanning salon, any more than someone selling cigarettes to kids. There are plenty of places to work and I'd love to see tanning salons go out of business because they couldn't find anyone to work there. Nothing good comes from tanning. Period. That is why I wrote this book. You don't need to go to med school or Google WebMD or ask your mother. You just stay far away from tanning salons. (See: https://www.cdc.gov/cancer/skin/basic_info/indoor_tanning.htm)

During the baroque period, being overweight was seen as an identifier of wealth (think of Rembrandt's paintings of naked, overweight men and women). People who had money had food and food made them fat, and hence the cultural idea that fat was beautiful. Similarly, today we believe that having a tan somehow signals popularity, coolness, attractiveness and status. Nothing could be further from the truth, and one day, future generations will ask themselves why government agencies allowed human cancer ovens to even exist.

To be completely clear and fair, every bronzed beauty doesn't fall into the category of stupid. Far from it. It is possible that they use a spray or self-tanning cream, although they too have questionable health effects. I will forgive people for vanity, but not for insanity.

If you must use your brain to learn more or challenge my position, then take a gander at the Skin Cancer Foundation's blog where real people tell their stories of tanning that turned deadly. Buckle up. It's not pretty. (See: https://blog.skincancer.org/2017/11/09/melanoma-bucket-list/)

I think you got the point. Grab a hat and let's move on.

CHAPTER THIRTEEN

ORAL HEALTH

A GOOD SMILE AND fresh breath can do a lot to help a hookup. According to that titan of medical research, Match.com, more than half of singles ranked teeth as the most important characteristic about a potential date in a survey of 5,500 unattached people. Now, it doesn't say perfect straight teeth, but rather just *teeth*. Not everyone has perfect teeth, nor do they need to spend a bunch of money to make them perfect. There is no health benefit related to perfectly straight teeth. But when it comes to clean teeth and gums, the results are clear. Bad oral health brings with it equally bad breath, which should be enough of a brainless reason to brush.

But bad breath is the absolute tip of the iceberg when it comes to bad brushing and flossing. What completely blows my mind about this health habit is that it has been taught to most people since before they were potty trained.

Brushing when you wake up and before bedtime is a more powerfully ingrained routine than praying before dinner, yet millions of people disregard it. (Hmmm, I wonder if the same people who don't wash their hands, don't brush their teeth?) They must literally think that their *breath doesn't* stink, and that their teeth repel plaque. They must also think that somehow they transcend the laws of disease. They must believe that even though they don't care for their teeth, they won't get nasty diseases, tooth loss and gum rot.

Truthfully, it never took talking about gum disease and plaque buildup to motivate me to brush. Maybe that's because I had never seen a disfiguring gum disease. I just obeyed my mother. Sadly, now I have seen the pictures and it is horrifying. Like so many other diseases, it also includes preventable cancers. Gingivitis and periodontitis are the two most common gum diseases, and the former causes bleeding of the gums, while the later leads to tooth loss.

That's enough for me. I am smart enough to know that teeth are anchored into place by bone, and once that bone erodes, the teeth are falling out. I wish there was an easy way to help people temporarily experience the effects of tooth loss, like blindfolding someone to appreciate blindness. If you talk to anyone who has experienced it, you should listen well. It is horrible.

We take our teeth for granted. Those who experience tooth loss experience pain and discomfort and significant social stigma. Try getting a job without a tooth. People don't react well to people with a hole in their smile. You could be a PhD physicist and people would assume that you hadn't graduated high school if you have one or more visible teeth missing, fair or not. For those who are financially able to afford false teeth, bridges and dentures, you will hear endless stories of embarrassment, inconvenience and significant stress related to caring for and maintaining them.

Fortunately, brushing is super easy and super brainless. It removes food that would otherwise fester in our mouth like the nasty, expired jar of spaghetti sauce in the back of your refrigerator. None of us like looking at someone with food in their teeth or at yellow buildup between their teeth. It's gross. Years of it is beyond gross.

It is obvious that leaving bacteria painted across your teeth can't be a good thing, and lots of scientific studies support it. What's worse is that gum and mouth diseases make simple brushing difficult and carry nasty smells. If foul breath motivates you to brush, then do it.

So, what's your *real* risk? Well, I am going to share what Delta Dental says about a few things that constitutes an increased level of risk for oral health problems such as decay, infection and cancer. Apparently, you're at higher risk of oral health problems if you:

- **Are a woman having hormonal changes.** *(As if hot flashes weren't enough.)* For women, hormonal changes around their period, menopause, and during pregnancy can cause inflamed gums (gingivitis). If left untreated, it can develop into a more serious gum disease called periodontitis.

- **Use tobacco.** *(Surprise, surprise.)* People who use tobacco, whether they smoke or chew, have a higher risk of the severe gum disease called periodontitis, and tooth loss. Tobacco users are also at high risk of cancers of the mouth, tongue, throat, and lips.

- **Drink alcohol.** *(I didn't know this.)* People who drink alcohol have a higher risk of oral cancers, especially if they are heavy drinkers.

- **Have certain diseases.** Health conditions such as diabetes, anemia, Sjögren's syndrome, cancer, hyperthyroidism, and HIV/AIDS can cause many oral health problems. People with these conditions are at higher risk for issues such as infections from yeast, fungus, or bacteria, plus tooth decay and gum disease. *(This is a significant reason to stay healthy. Disease begets disease. Multiple chronic conditions characterize millions of Americans.)*

- **Taking certain medications.** Many medications can cause dry mouth, a condition where there isn't enough saliva in the mouth. Saliva helps prevents infection, gum disease, and tooth decay. *(Who would have guessed that your saliva protects you from tooth decay?)* Dry mouth puts you at higher risk for these problems. Some medication for allergies, high blood pressure, and depression can cause dry mouth as well. Some narcotic pain medications used after injury or surgery can also cause dry mouth. Fortunately, they make mouthwash and other products to combat dry mouth. Ask your pharmacist or dentist. It's a big deal but super easy to combat.

- **Are an older adult.** As we age, our mouths can produce less saliva. Many older adults are on medications that can cause dry mouth, and our gums tend to recede or get lower along the tooth line as we age. This can expose the roots of the teeth, which don't have the hard layer of enamel to protect them. Root tooth decay can be a more common problem among older adults. Oral cancers are also more common in people ages fifty-five and older.

- **Have poor dental hygiene.** Not brushing and flossing daily can cause plaque to build up and harden onto teeth. This can cause gum disease, inflamed gums that are red and bleed easily. Untreated, this can turn into periodontitis and even tooth loss.

- **Have oral sex with a person who has HPV.** Human papillomavirus (HPV) has been shown to cause cancers, and it can cause oral cancers from sexual contact. A brainless strategy is simply to get tested along with your partner. A positive diagnosis doesn't mean that you have to break up, it will just inform your behavior. There are plenty of walk-in testing clinics, if you are embarrassed to ask your doctor about sexually transmitted diseases such as HPV or HIV. Consider sticking with your kisser until you get the test results, my friends.

- **Are a man.** Men have twice the risk of oral cancers as women. Go figure.

- **Spend a lot of time in the sun or use a tanning booth.** Cancer of the lips is more common in people who have a lot of exposure to UV rays, such as in sunlight or tanning booths.

- **Have a close family member with poor oral health.** Unfortunately, some oral health problems may be linked to genes. This means that getting more tooth decay or gum problems may run in families. You're more at risk for oral problems if your family has a history of them. While genetics are an unavoidable risk, you can beat your genetic disposition by working harder. If you have a history of heart disease or alcoholism, you have to be more vigilant and more proactive to beat it before it beats you. It is relatively easy to do, but you have to be aware and conscientious.

- **Use illegal drugs.** Use of cannabis (weed) has the same risks as the use of tobacco, a greater chance of periodontitis and tooth loss. You're also at higher risk of oral cancer. Using methamphetamine can cause severe tooth decay, periodontitis, and the loss of many teeth, also known as *meth mouth.* Heroin, opium, cocaine, and MDMA (Ecstasy) can lead to tooth decay and gum disease.

- **Have poor nutrition.** Not getting the right vitamins and minerals in your diet can cause the body to have problems fighting infection. Model good nutritional health to your kids and it will eliminate a million issues down the road.

- **Have stress.** Stress also harms the body's ability to fight infection. This can turn small oral health problems into big oral health problems.

A few years ago, a presenter at a health conference asked the audience of health professionals whether they brushed their teeth to improve their breath. Ninety-nine percent of the audience raised hands. They believed that brushing improved their breath. According to the presenter, however, flossing is the real breath freshener. My research revealed that the verdict is still out on the subject, but I did learn that used floss smells. Yep, smelling that tiny string never crossed my mind, but apparently it smells pretty bad. Many believe that is because it has reached the abyss between your teeth, two millimeters below your gum, where aging bacteria live. Whether or not this is correct, it seems plausible to me to eradicate that stench and keep flossing.

Let me be clear. Whether flossing helps prevent disease or not is irrelevant to me. Removing food (and sticky plaque) that my toothbrush failed to reach simply makes sense. More than 700 different bacteria are said to live in your mouth and can colonize below the gum and cause significant health issues. Hello? *Colonize below the gum.* Think termites in your house. You don't see them. No one does. Until you see the damage that they cause. That's what gum disease is all about. By the time your gums start to bleed, you are screwed. So just remember, when you put the floss in and pull out stuff that is stuck to it, that's a good thing. Get the food out of your mouth, hook or by crook. Period.

Finally, I love the sign in my sister's bathroom that reads, "Only floss the teeth you want to keep." That sums it up perfectly for me.

CHAPTER FOURTEEN

METAL-HEALTH DETECTORS

MOST OF US DON'T think twice about going through a metal detector at the airport or public event because we see it as a relatively small inconvenience to protect us from someone blowing up our plane. Well, that's what I am talking about when it comes to your health. You don't want some actual terrorist cell to blow up your colon or liver or pancreas or breast or prostate. We are talking about the same thing—terrorist detection. Disease detection. Death prevention. Fortunately, getting screened for diseases is typically as innocuous as walking through a metal detector.

I can hear you objecting, wanting to remind me that I'm not a woman so I haven't felt the pain of a mammogram. I can also hear the male readers *asking me* to bend over for a prostate exam. Sure, there can be discomfort, *but not nearly as much* as enduring chemotherapy or radiation. Give me a break. Just ask a cancer survivor if they wish their cancer had been detected earlier. How about someone who lost their parent or child because they never got screened.

Of course, today it's vogue to talk about how medical screenings (and even airport screenings) actually *cause cancer* from the radiation. I sit in amazement because we have finally made it to an era of scientific breakthroughs that can catch things before they kill you, yet people would rather do what? Hope? Cross their fingers? Chant? Seriously, what are the alternatives? Wheat grass shots? Get real and get screened. Let's agree to silence the slightest objection to routine health screenings.

The next time someone goes to the doctor with a chest cough, should they turn down a chest X-ray and just keep hacking and hoping that it will just all go away? Of course not. How many people with chronic migraines should just keep popping ibuprofen instead of getting an MRI? And when it comes to airports, everyone can talk about the potential harm of metal detectors, but few would prefer that TSA stopped screening passengers. Believe me, I've been patted down by TSA, and I'm not willing to bet their hands against a metal detector, ever!

It's interesting and even useful to discuss the possible ramifications of such screening tools, and I think we need to continue to search for safer and safer methods. Trust me, the industry is continually trying to improve the screening technology to reduce risk and create less invasive procedures if for no other reason than to sell more machines, make more money and screen more people. But in the meantime, let's use what we've got.

I want your brainless reaction to be, "Yes Doctor. Do it. Screen me. Tell me when and where." And if your doctor isn't telling you to get screened (as some don't), please ask them for a mammogram or colonoscopy or prostate exam or eye exam or liver scan or ultrasound. That's *your* job. Ask for a life-saving detection of anything that may be lurking below the surface, anything that concerns you.

Let me be clear. I'm not talking about just blindly getting body scans willy-nilly or following the marketing of every electromagnetic medical device. Nor am I talking about treatment. Treatment for illness is far from brainless. The verdict is out on *all kinds* of disease treatments, *but discovering the problem is brainless.* I think everyone is happy that car manufacturers now have diagnostic tools that illuminate a check-engine light when things are about to go wrong. It sure beats getting surprised when the water pump or carbon monoxide sensor or alternator fails and leaves you on the side of the road or careening out of control. Sure, plenty of people just keep driving when that check-engine light comes on, but at least they have been warned. You might not choose to fix the problem in your liver or colon, but you sure want to know what's going on.

There are definitely cases where a screening of some kind had some ill effect. But there are literally millions of living human beings who would be dead if it wasn't for early detection.

My wife is not a lover of pills or doctor visits, but recently she recounted the story of a family member who had zero symptoms until they discovered that tongue cancer had been growing for two years and would soon kill her. An annual exam *would have* caught it early, but she had stopped getting her annual exams. Don't want to wait for symptoms to act.

While family history is a critically important justification for people to get checked, the CDC reports that most people who get cancer have *zero* family history of cancer. *Zero!* If you have family history, you are at an increased risk, but lack of family history means nothing. So, everyone needs to get screened.

It is easy to discuss the topic of screening from a theoretical or academic standpoint until you are face-to-face with a cancer patient. A very close friend of mine recently died from bladder cancer. After a few years of remission following surgery and radiation, it came back. They caught it of course because he was being monitored, but what struck me was his comments about his change in perspective. He was the single most intellectual friend I have ever had. But as soon as the cancer came into his life, he renounced all skepticism about screenings.

Disease is the great equalizer. It cripples our intellect as well as our physical bodies. Suddenly the discussions of to screen or not to screen become irrelevant. The moment you learn that you have cancer, you simply want the doctors to use every resource to save your life.

Remember, not all screenings involve radiation, metal objects or rectal cameras. Self-exams are wildly effective at detecting trouble. Breast and testicular self-exams, for example, are highly effective methods of detection and are highly underutilized for some inexplicable reason. Most people take a shower once a day, which is the best time to probe your body. If you have a significant other that you like to shower or sleep with, I'm sure they'd be happy to help.

Full body skin exams are another example of a non-invasive scan. It consists of a dermatologist simply looking at your body. If they find an unusual mole, they might whip out a magnifying glass, but that is it. Another close friend of mine survived melanoma simply because his wife detected an unusually dark mole on his bottom. That's a place he couldn't see by himself, and his wife saved his life by just paying attention.

Recently, I read about a woman who was strongly opposed to vaccinations. One day she contracted whooping cough, a contagious bacterial disease that often affects children and is characterized by convulsive coughing. When she ended up giving it to her unvaccinated child, who nearly died, her opinion about vaccinations changed overnight.

Listen to your doctor and use advances in science and technology to be proactive with the care of your body and those around you. We all need to avail ourselves of the tools that science has developed, from scanners to pharmaceuticals. Not all are created equal and some have side effects. Nevertheless, it is important to weigh those side effects against death and disability.

The famous journalist Joan Lunden tells the story of how she got a mammogram and it was all clear. She and her family literally celebrated for ten minutes in the doctor's office until they moved her across the hall and ordered an ultrasound to confirm the results. Just a few minutes later, the doctor said she had breast cancer. That's because not all tests are equal. Not all tests see the same things. She now recommends that *all women* should ask for an ultrasound regardless of the report from their mammogram. Listen to your doctor, listen to your friends, but don't rely on them. Don't rely on Google or WebMD either. Research the topic, collect data and then ask questions. It is not easy. It can be downright confusing and overwhelming, but no one will be a better advocate for your body than yourself.

Another very close friend was diagnosed with colon cancer. She had been diligent to get her colon tested regularly in her thirties because her father died of colon cancer at age thirty-nine. Well, sure enough she got colon cancer just like her dad. In fact, she was stage four. Like most people, her doctor gave her the conventional wisdom of chemo and radiation. She and her husband talked about it and asked about survival rates and started researching alternatives treatments. They discovered mistletoe therapy being used in Germany. It is not FDA approved in the US, so they had to find a doctor who would be willing to administer it for her. Ten years later, she is still alive and still cancer free. But it didn't stop there. She wanted to make this therapy available to other cancer patients in the US, so she started her own foundation and raised over $300,000. She then convinced Johns Hopkins to launch the very first clinical trial in the US (Check out her nonprofit at www.BelieveBig.org). She has now helped thousands of patients beat cancer.

When I say that you must be your own advocate, I mean it. When I say that you should take advantage of every kind of screening, surgery, therapy, pill, prayer, I mean it. Remember, you are not just fighting for your life, you are fighting for *your best* life. You might die fighting, but you might also get to live to see your kid graduate. You might die fighting, but maybe you won't have to suffer in a wheelchair for the last fifteen years of your life. You might die fighting, but at the very least you will inspire, educate and lead others.

Recently, my work with the CDC involved helping patients who were diagnosed with triple negative breast cancer, a rare disease that doesn't respond to typical treatments. The purpose of the work was to help patients decide on a path of treatment. A lot of patients get so overwhelmed with the mere diagnosis of cancer that they are mentally paralyzed and choose to do nothing. *Nothing.* They literally get zero treatment for their cancer and suffer terribly simply because they cannot decide what to do. Sometimes, under life-threatening circumstances, we have to work really hard, but if you are frozen and unable to do the work, at least listen to your doctor. That's the brainless part.

If you do nothing else that I recommend in this book, please get checked, get scanned, get screened, get immunized, get poked, prodded and protected. Take advantage of the world-class health detectors that can discover what you can't see or feel.

CHAPTER FIFTEEN

SEX ON THE BEACH

I HAVE TO SAY that I'm a big fan of the *sex on the beach* cocktail, but the real thing is a whole lot better for you. Fortunately, everyone can garner the health benefits of sex, whether they are on the beach or in their bed.

Consider the acronym for sex on the beach (SOTB) as a brainless quick-reference-guide to achieving romantic, *healthy* sex, no matter what the location.

First, you begin to want **SEX**. It all starts with the desire. You become physically and psychologically attracted to your lover. You are feeling amorous. Chemicals are being released in your body and drawing you to each other.

Second, you consciously decide to do things to specifically turn **ON** your lover. You are doing what you know he/she likes and what comes naturally in the heat of the moment. You have prepared for this moment and your behaviors are specific, targeted turn-ons.

Third, your lover is **THE** focus of your attention and vice versa. They are your only concern. They are at the center of your universe. Their body and emotions. You don't compare yourself to anyone else because you are focused on the *other* person. There are no cellphone or email distractions to compete with them.

Finally, you are on the **BEACH**, metaphorically. Your surroundings are naturally romantic and conducive for sex. You are alone. No one is around to disturb you or interrupt you. Your environment is perfect for intimacy.

Not all sex has SOTB ingredients, but when possible, it's a great standard to shoot for. Sadly, it wasn't until the famous researchers Masters and Johnson officially made the study of sexuality and sexual behavior downright vogue in 1957 that people permitted themselves to delve into the health implications of this incredibly healthy, yet primal act. Since then, there have been thousands of studies and theories about the *health of sex* as well as what constitutes *healthy sex*. From intercourse to masturbation to oral sex to orgasms, sexual activity has largely been declared healthy, inside healthy contexts.

I know that you are probably thinking that you can't wait to tell your partner that you need to have more sex to improve your overall health. It's certainly worth a try, but note that not all sex is created equal and therefore all sex does not bear the same health benefits.

SETTING THE RELATIONAL STAGE

First, good form is critical to obtaining the greatest health benefits from sex. Healthy sex transcends the physical and includes the mental, emotional and even spiritual. Therefore, a *solid relational foundation* will always deliver the maximum health benefits. In other words, one-night stands don't meet the health criteria discussed in this book.

Nevertheless, as healthful as sex can be in strong relationships, it is often described by some as casual or meaningless, routine or boring. Some people use the words obligatory and even painful to describe their sexual experience. Fortunately, none of this need be the case if a few brainless behaviors are incorporated into intimate relationships.

Any person in a committed relationship knows that romance and respect are powerful aphrodisiacs. In other words, those who bring flowers, take out the trash, dress well, smell good, cook or buy dinner, do the dishes, open the door or open their wallet, are far more likely to have healthy sex because all of those things also build healthy relationships.

Therefore, the most brainless sexual behavior is simply the Golden Rule. You don't have to be a relationship counselor or a sex therapist. Just look in the mirror and ask yourself what you want in a sexual relationship, such as desire, passion, appreciation, value, admiration, respect and even a fantasy or two. It is no more difficult than that. Lead by example. Of course, that is step one. Model chivalry or sexiness or spontaneity or romance. Go over the top if that's what you want and what you value.

The next step is to convey those things to your partner by delivering *intentional actions followed by genuine words*. In other words, start with behaviors and then follow up with sentiment. Not the other way around. Words can be cheap, but actions require effort. Fortunately, the effort can still be brainless. You can buy the jewelry or the perfume or the golf club. You can book the restaurant or pick the movie. Words that are authentic, on the other hand, can be more difficult, especially if time has passed and you don't typically stare into each other's eyes and share your feelings. Words require vulnerability, and actions set the perfect stage for words to follow. *Loving words naturally follow loving actions.*

So, start with what you *can do,* whether it is coming home early, putting down the cell phone, closing the computer or simply listening to the other person. Fill the tank with gas, grab some flowers while picking up the milk, buy a greeting card or prepare the bedroom for sex including candles, music, lighting, sheets, etc.

Then comes the truly brainless part. Make it a habit. Stop by the florist every Friday on the way home. Buy different flowers each time. You will surprise your partner with something new and also learn his or her favorites. Buy a greeting card every time you go to the grocery store and a book of stamps. Take your lover's car to the carwash every Tuesday. Pick up a Starbucks gift card when you are getting your coffee. The key is to have this stuff on hand. Slip a gift card or greeting card, or homemade card, into his/her computer from time to time as a surprise. Buy a stack of sticky notes. Stick sweet messages on the bathroom mirror or the car window or the rearview mirror. I could write a whole book about these simple, brainless, inexpensive acts that will make men and women swoon.

People like to know that you are thinking of them. Reread that. It's that simple. Whatever you do, make sure the other person knows that you are thinking about them. Phones are great for sending text messages in the middle of meetings, but it is also the easiest thing to do. We are not aiming for ease. We are aiming for things that are *easy to remember* but impactful. Brainless actions still require effort because effort generates results.

Sometimes these beautiful acts of love do not generate more sex or different sex, or right now sex, but they certainly don't hurt. They prepare the body, heart and mind for intimacy. Plus, there's no reason you can't spice up your loving, brainless acts to more explicitly communicate your interests. Include a sexy picture in your greeting card or buy a lingerie gift card instead of a coffee card. Write sexy compliments on your sticky notes or schedule date nights complete with reservations and a babysitter. The bottom line is that performing regular acts of romance, kindness, appreciation and admiration will warm the waters for intimacy. You *model* the behavior you would like, then *augment with words.*

There is a great book by Gary Chapman called *The Five Love Languages.* It is a super easy read and a critical breakthrough in relationships. You could be giving your spouse lots of gifts, but really all she/he values is time with you. Similarly, you could be spending lots of sacrificial time and all he/she wants are words of affirmation or gifts. We have different love languages that uniquely melt our hearts.

If your idea of great sex includes something like bondage or role playing, then you will likely have to supplement your actions with a good deal of dialogue. It's not enough to buy the handcuffs or maid costume. You need to create an environment of safety and honest communication. Then discuss your desires and show the other person that you are willing to buy the goods, set the mood and create a fun experience. Sadly, a friend of mine orchestrated a super sexy evening by renting a private *red room of pain* because of his wife's obsession with the *Fifty Shades of Grey* trilogy. He surprised her, and when they arrived, she was completely freaked out and not into the idea of bondage at all. A little conversation would have gone a long way and saved a chunk of change. Sometimes the reason fantasies are attractive is because they are fantasies.

DEMONSTRATION AND COMMUNICATION

Too many long-term relationships and marriages get into a sexual rut because they have established false perceptions about who the other person is and what they would or wouldn't want. I've talked to countless men and women who repeat the words, "He/she would never do that." That's where it stops. It's hard to be vulnerable and tell someone what you want in the bedroom. It's incredibly hard. Sometimes, it can be easier to do the asking. In other words, ask them what turns them on, what they would like to try or be super specific that your question only requires a yes or no answer. While it can still be scary to answer such questions, they will simply be responding to you instead of bringing up the topic. Typically, that person will then ask you a similar question and, *violà*, you are having a sexy conversation.

Strangely, after two people have created a safe space, full of trust and grace in a committed relationship, sexual conversation and experimentation can become the hardest areas to traverse or transcend. Maybe because of culture, or religion. Who knows and who cares, but it is pervasive and damaging. Sexless marriages are analogous to disease because they can cause major ill-health effects from depression to obesity, to say nothing of increasing the risk for excitement substitutes such as alcohol, drugs, gambling, shopping or infidelity. Sex connects us. It improves intimacy, and when *sexual intimacy* is *not* practiced in a committed relationship that is intended for intimacy, it can lead to anger, depression, rejection and loss of self-worth.

When you start a relationship, sexual preferences are rarely the first thing you talk about over a candlelight dinner (although it's a great idea). Sex can often just evolve out of passion and opportunity, but after lots of movies and dinners and meeting the parents, let alone a career and a few kids, the sex that marked the relationship in the early days may be collecting cobwebs. It's the focus of countless sitcom jokes about marriage but never very funny in real life.

Dylan Selterman, a social psychologist at the University of Maryland, says that having an honest conversation with your partner about your relationship is critical. "Doing everything right," he says, "can mean many different things. It could be the case that you think things are going very, very well, but in your partner's mind maybe not so much. It could be the case that there's room for improvement or that partners have not been on the same page." Few understand the importance (and ease) of demonstrating and communicating exactly what they want. When a man brings home a ribbon-topped box of lingerie, he may be saying that he wants to see his wife in those panties or teddy. He might also simply be buying her a romantic gift that she might not buy for herself. *Doing and saying* need to go together, especially in the land of intimacy where vulnerability and emotions run high.

So, take a deep breath and talk about your sex life, but do so with plenty of love-filled actions that precede the conversation. Express yourself within the context of demonstratively generous, thoughtful and romantic actions. Remember, too, that actions don't require feelings; feelings will typically follow. We don't have to feel romantic or appreciated to buy flowers or send a card or cook a special meal. Just do it. Brainless, automatic and even systematic.

I like to say, *the more thoughtless the thoughtful act, the more appreciative the appreciation.* When it becomes second nature for us to do sweet things like pouring a drink for someone after work or buying a favorite food at the grocery, sweetness gets ingrained into the fabric of that person. It becomes part of their character and pays exponential dividends. Just imagine one of your friends telling about how Ted vacuums Tina's car every Tuesday or how Julie buys Jim a new brand of gin whenever she travels on business. They just do it, and soon, the actions mellow into a glow of appreciation, respect and mutual love. *Tiny acts of love do wonders for quelling tiny acts of irritation.* Never forget that. Millions of stupid arguments that typically prevent intimacy could be avoided by simple acts of love.

What's not always obvious is that the more often you have sex, the more likely you (and your partner) will actually want to keep doing it. Physically and emotionally. It's the epitome of brainless. It starts to become a hardwired desire like muscle memory.

THERAPEUTIC SEX

Years ago, I went to my first (and last) hot yoga session. There were tiny windows all sealed up near the ceiling, and the room felt like it was 1,000 degrees. I sweated like never before. After dripping all over the mat, moaning like a child and feeling my ligaments stretch beyond natural limits, I finally felt like I could wrap my leg around my head and scratch my nose. I felt like a rubber band. That's the kind of relaxation some people get from sex. Stress disappears. It has been rung out of them and suddenly the things that seemed so important in life strangely feel far less important. Typically, physical aches and pains disappear as well. The oxytocin, dopamine and other chemicals that are released lead to a new level of patience and peace and feeling of well-being.

A long sexual workout leaves both people listless on the bed, or a ravaging quickie can be equally gratifying. Neither is better than the other when it comes to physical and emotional health. One person's gold standard isn't any more healthful than another. Any expression of love in a relationship provides plenty of healthy benefits, far beyond the sweaty palms and heightened breathing.

Sex is a natural pain reliever. I love telling people, "Instead of saying *no to sex* because of a headache, say *yes to sex because of a headache!*" One study in *Clinical Neurology* February 19, 2013, found that sexual activity can lead to partial or complete relief of headache in some migraine and cluster-headache patients. Sexual activity also releases pain-reducing hormones that have been found to help reduce or block back and leg pain, as well as pain from menstrual cramps and arthritis.

Sex reduces disease risk. WebMD also reports that sex improves your immune system, lowers blood pressure, and decreases heart attack risk. (JAMA. 2004;291(13):1578-1586. doi:10.1001/jama.291.13.1578.) It also helps with women's bladder control and reduces stress while improving sleep. (See: https://www.webmd.com/sex-relationships/guide/sex-and-health#3)

While the conclusions are inconclusive (don't you love that), studies have linked male ejaculation with a reduction in prostate cancer. One 2004 study, reported in *European Urology*, was followed up in 2016 and reported that men who ejaculated at least twenty-one times a month had a reduced risk for prostate cancer compared to men who only ejaculated four-to-seven times a month. In 2008 another study asserted that the linkage was only attributable in men over fifty. In the end, the relationship between the prostate and ejaculation still needs more research, but I'm sure millions of men will be happy to sign up for the study.

Best of all, a 2006 report in *Biological Psychology* revealed that men who made love at least twice a week were 45 percent less likely to develop heart disease than those who did so once a month or less. (See: Biol Psychol. 2006 Feb;71(2):214-22.) That tidbit is worth the price of this book.

Sex makes you smarter. According to *Psychology Today*, sex can even make you smarter. It reports that sex can change your brain chemistry in ways that increase your cognitive capacity. A study published in the *Personality and Social Psychology Bulletin* found that even just thinking about a sexual encounter can enhance analytic skills. Another study on rats indicated that sexually-active rodents had more neurons in the part of their brain responsible for the storage of memories than non-active rats. The neurons decreased after sexual activity stopped.

In related research on the female orgasm, it was found that sexual climax activates as many as thirty areas of the brain. Blood flows in, carrying a surge of nutrients and oxygen to brain cells. By contrast, popular brain games such as Sudoku or crosswords engage only a handful at best. (See: https://www.psychologytoday.com/us/blog/the-mating-game/201602/7-compelling-reasons-have-more-sex)

Sex makes you look and feel younger. If making you smarter wasn't enough good news, apparently, sex can make you look and feel younger. Yep. You need to bookmark this chapter.

Americans spend billions of dollars every year on chemicals and procedures and snake-oil potions in the pursuit of youth. But according to *Psychology Today*, a British study found that having regular sex can make both men and women *look* between five and ten years younger. Intercourse causes the release of human growth hormone, which sets off a range of biological reactions with the ultimate effect of making the skin appear more elastic and smoother. Sex also triggers the release of estrogen, which improves the quality of hair and skin. The lead researcher of this study previously demonstrated that while mental and physical activity is the most important factor for retaining one's youth, regular sex was a close second.

As I've discussed, sexual activity in the context of a committed relationship that is emotionally safe and secure is truly chock full of health. That emotional security allows the body to release healthy hormones such as oxytocin and vasopressin. Oxytocin is often nicknamed the *cuddle hormone* for the obvious reason. Like dopamine, oxytocin is produced by the hypothalamus and released in large quantities during sex. It makes you feel exceptionally good. It draws you to your partner. It solidifies and codifies and reinforces the fact that you are together and that you are wanted.

If you want to know more about vasopressin, Google it because it is far too complex for this book and far less understood scientifically than oxytocin. Nevertheless, scientists think that it may lead to pairing or bonding, which in the context of a committed relationship is awesome.

I don't want to get into all the science, but trust me, there are plenty of articles to keep you awake at night (when you should be having sex) if you really want to delve into the science of sex.

The emotional health benefits of sex are often even more important than the physical health aspects. That is because as human beings we crave connection. Of course, family and friends are essential to emotional and relational health; however, one can experience uniquely specialized health effects by connecting sexually with a soulmate, lover or spouse. Such relationships include feelings of security, value, worth and meaning that are different than in other relational contexts. These feelings validate us and remind us that someone chooses to be with us in an intimate way that signals a heightened sense of trust and connection and safety.

ANOTHER SIDE OF SEX

As healthful as sex can be under the right circumstances, it can also be one of the most dangerous, anti-health activities on the planet.

In addition to having deadly physical consequences from disease and infection, it can produce unfathomable mental and emotional harm.

It can be full of anxiety, guilt and endless regret. That's *even if you don't* get an STD, an unwanted pregnancy or a lifetime prescription for herpes medication. I remember a woman who told me that her STD wasn't that big a deal because she just took medication when she had a breakout. Are you kidding me? When was the last genital breakout that wasn't a *big deal*? Try having a herpes breakout on your next beach vacation or anniversary.

People cease to amaze me. I'm all for minimizing your pain and suffering, but let's not mask the ugly reality of the dangers of sex. In fact, sex with strangers, hookups, dating-app-sex, prostitutes or one-night stands have a high probability of danger. That's because those who engage in sexual promiscuity are typically rockin' and rollin' with other people who are *also* promiscuous. If you haven't taken a course in statistics, don't worry. It simply means that you are increasing your chances of disaster the more times you roll the dice.

If I fly once a year, I have a statistically lower chance of being killed on an airplane crash than someone who flies every week. It's as simple as that. When you are screwing people who are screwing lots of other people, you are increasing your chances that you are going to get screwed, with an STD or worse.

Believe it or not, there are far more serious emotional, mental and spiritual maladies associated with casual sex than just the physical ones. Guilt over lack of judgement (especially if cheating is involved) can haunt people for a lifetime. Anxiety, generated from wondering if you have a disease or an unwanted pregnancy on the way, can ravage the mind and create emotions that in turn affect the physical body. Never forget that the mind and body are symbiotic systems. One impacts the other and vice versa.

Fears of being discovered or exploited on social media can be truly terrifying and completely life altering. Such social media scenarios are portrayed in movies, TV dramas and sitcoms, but the way they play out in real life is not for the faint of heart and possesses debilitating consequences.

Having sex for you might simply be a physical release, but for the other person it can mean much more psychologically. And rarely will that surface until after the fact. Feelings of responsibility or obligation can also result in rash decisions to either move forward in an unhealthy relationship or pull out of an otherwise healthy one.

My friend and his fiancée were in an exclusive and committed relationship when she found out that she had HPV after one year of dating. The woman called my friend and told him she was breaking off the engagement so that he would not be at risk for getting HPV. Fortunately, he convinced her otherwise and today the virus has left her body and they are happily married. The point is that the emotional impact of sexually transmitted diseases can lead to unfathomable consequences.

I read about a man who spent twenty-five years wondering if he had fathered a daughter by a high school hookup. They didn't have the ability to conduct a DNA test back then and so he lived with confusion, fear and guilt. After all those years, the mother contacted him and asked him for a DNA test, which confirmed he had no connection to the girl. One night in high school caused twenty-five long years of suffering by all parties.

I love to remind people that it is a gift that is not easily given away. In other words, all consensual sex involves *some degree of effort*. Therefore, it can be closely held, hidden in the vault and only reserved for that special person given the code. It can be protected and cherished and relished. Then it becomes elevated to the point of something healthful to the soul, not cheapened or minimized.

Don't get me wrong; it doesn't have to be prim and proper (unless that's how you like it), but it should be personal, relational, special, reserved. Every culture in history has gone through a stage of free love and never has it become a best practice. It's amazing. Even the Woodstock music festival, free-love mantra didn't become the norm.

Instead, for thousands of years, across geographies and cultures and languages and religions, people have signed onto the idea that human intimacy is intimate. It is reserved for relationship.

MORE GOOD NEWS

Sex should not define intimacy. Intimacy is the goal because it is much broader than just sex. A woman might be on her period or intercourse might be painful. A man might be dealing with erectile dysfunction or simply exhausted from stress. Both people can still reap many of the same health benefits from sex, through other forms of intimate contact, like hugging and kissing and touching.

According to Dr. Joseph Mercola (Mercola.com), hugging is known to lower levels of stress hormones like cortisol. He reports that hugging also activates the orbitofrontal cortex in your brain, which is linked to feelings of reward and compassion. A ten-second hug a day can lead to biochemical and physiological reactions in your body that can significantly improve your health. So, at very least get generous with your hugs and kisses.

CHAPTER SIXTEEN

DIET—NOT DIETING

FOOD IS THE MOST important—and arguably the most controversial—topic related to your health. I cannot turn on the TV without someone spouting off about beets or bone broth or juicing. Believe me, I've tried them all. I've tried paleo. I've tried keto. I've tried Whole 30 and I've tried Raw. I've even tried the grapefruit and black coffee diet.

Some helped me lose weight. Some helped me sleep better. Some helped me have more energy. The problem is that each has detractors, and none are *brainless*. When on these fad diets, I was always wondering what I was doing to my body. How was it affecting my liver or my spleen or my kidneys or my heart? Moreover, each had a high or low level of difficulty related to maintaining it. If I traveled or went to a restaurant (or decided to eat with my family), I was pretty much screwed.

At the end of the day, I was doomed simply because I was pursuing *a diet*, instead of refining *my diet*. For the purposes of this book, the word *diet* is not something you *go on* for a time; nor is it a weight-loss strategy. Rather, diet refers to what you eat, week in and week out, good or bad. You can have a steady *diet* of cheeseburgers and chips, or a *diet* of celery and watercress. It's not about *a* diet but rather about *your* diet. In fact, I want you to never *go on a diet* again. I want you to banish that useless phrase from your grammar completely. Instead, I want you to *have a diet* of delicious health and nutrition.

Always remember, *the healthier your diet is, the healthier you will be.* Super brainless. Plus, if you refine your daily diet, your body will respond without feeling deprived or restrained. Over time, your taste buds will change, and you will start to crave healthy food and your former diet of junk will taste too sweet or too salty or give you a stomachache. Your body will adapt. It's amazing.

Ok, so how do you do this? Get ready for two completely brainless approaches to food that are worth sharing with everyone you know.

1. If it is grown on a tree or in the ground, **eat it**.
    Fruits and vegetables. (Sorry, no weed or tobacco.)
2. If it has wings or fins, **eat it.** Fish and chicken.

I call it the *F&V/F&C Diet.* That's easy to remember. Say it. It is kind of catchy, and the acronym kind of rhymes. *Fruits & Vegetables / Fish & Chicken.* If you did nothing else in this book other than that, you'd be healthier in a matter of days. It's that powerful.

Fortunately, it's easy to shop for F&V/F&C items and easy to cook them. It's easy to order them on a menu. It's just super, stupid, simple, and if you stick to it, you will improve your metabolic numbers, lose weight and feel better. Plus, it is delicious. You can follow it for appetizers, entrees and even dessert. I considered writing a companion F&V/F&C cookbook, but there are already enough cookbooks in the world. Instead, if you like cookbooks, just flip through them and pick out the recipes that consist of F&V/F&C.

If you focus on these four food areas, you will never run out of options, your meals won't get boring and you will almost always find something on the restaurant menu to order. Most importantly, you won't feel like you are punishing or depriving yourself. That is the key. Punishment and deprivation is never connected to brainlessness. Punishment and deprivation is why fad diets don't work. They are not sustainable. They are not fulfilling or fun. You are always aware of how hungry you are or how long you have until the suffering is over.

Conversely, F&V/F&C is always yummy, and you can always supplement if you want. Have a steak if you want or even a Pop Tart® every now and then, but the goal with F&V/F&C is to train your brain to go there automatically. You see berries on the menu, you order them. You see chicken, you cook it. You see fish, you put it in your cart. You see any kind of veggies, you get them, store them, cook them, order them, eat them and repeat.

Sure, it is better if you avoid French fries or fried catfish or even fried Brussels sprouts, but you get the idea. This is a brainless hack. It is designed to push you in the right direction and get you to second base. The nutrition in these foods will typically be better than foods devoid of such nutrition. Even when my salad is drenched in dressing, I'm still getting nutrients from my greens which I would not get at all if I ordered something without veggies. Once you master F&V/F&C, then you can refine the process.

Remember, you can have fish or chicken marinated in a million flavors and you can order your fish sautéed, grilled, blackened, fileted or whole. Sushi is my personal favorite. And your chicken certainly doesn't have to come from the Colonel. Today, chicken or fish tacos almost always comes with a grilled option. Even buffalo wings come grilled, dry rubbed or *lightly* battered. Practically every fish or chicken dish has a healthy version.

The same goes for veggies. Shred them, toss them, cook them, or eat them raw. Dip them or kabob them on the grill. Veggies make great appetizers and great side dishes. Gone are the days of Mom's nasty, canned, overcooked green beans. Gone are boiled potatoes (unless you like them that way) and gone are the days of celery and carrot sticks in your lunch box. Today, kung pow Brussels sprouts are served at the fanciest restaurants and carrots are pureed and sold as health-shots. Onions are skewered and pickled. Pickles are added to everything. There is simply no limit to the vegetable varieties. If you can't give up potato chips (yes, I know they are vegetables), try veggie chips such as beet chips, snap peas or green beans. They aren't much better, but I am asking you to re-orient your brain toward other veggies like sweet potatoes, peas and carrots.

I love these new dried snap peas that are chipotle and black-pepper flavored. Go figure. Or how about salt and vinegar, sweet-potato chips? Again, I know that they have about the same calories as potato chips and aren't optimum, but they steer you away from even *less healthy* snacks and they will help you fulfil your F&V/F&C mantra. Plus, because they are different, or come in smaller bags, or aren't as good for dipping in sour cream onion dip, you just might eat fewer of them.

I once overheard a kid say to his mother, "Strawberries are healthy because they are grown on trees." She corrected him, but who cares? He got the point that they didn't show up from a processing plant. They didn't come with a bunch of preservatives or chemicals in a jar or a can or a box.

Sure, fruits have loads of sugar, but it's not added or processed sugar. Of course, too many fruits can be problematic, so don't eat a pineapple for dinner and a bucket of strawberries for dessert. Sugar is a massive enemy, but fruit has fiber which your body loves (and most people don't get enough fiber). Too much fiber will either clog you up or clean you out depending on your body. If you eat too much fruit, you will soon be spending a lot of time on the toilet or have other discomfort that will teach you how to consume it smartly. In other words, don't worry about it. Your fruit intake will take care of itself.

You should also think of fruit as dessert. Whether they arrive straight off the tree, sliced up in a bowl, candied or dried, treat them like a *treat*, just like chocolate or cake, and you'll be good to go.

And, by the way, fruits and vegetables are seasonal. That means you should eat them in their season. Due to globalization and transportation, we can now eat strawberries 365 days a year if we want. But that's unnatural. That is not how nature produces them and not how the human body is designed to benefit from them. Therefore, stick to the seasons and you will improve your health while looking forward to seasonal recipes. I remember looking forward to foods in season, like peach pies and bowls of fresh cherries, strawberry jam, etc. Plus, eating fruit in season is a whole lot cheaper. It's brainless and fun.

Also, don't get too hung up on how your F&V/F&C foods are prepared when you are eating out at restaurants. Sure, they are cooked in butter. Sure, they come with oils and seasoning. Sure, you can request that they cook it a certain way, but that's far from brainless. Just accept that sometimes your food is going to be more healthy than other times, but if you stick to eating fruits and vegetables, fish and chicken, then you are going to be getting tons of protein, tons of Omega 3 fatty acids, tons of vitamins and tons of nutrients. Period.

You can play around with gluten all you want. Experiment with dairy. Enjoy your whole grains and probiotics and even your red meat, but if you really want to keep it simple and healthy and not get confused when you enter the grocery store or review the menu, stick to F&V/F&C.

I married a Peruvian. Apparently, *pollo las brasas* (Peruvian rotisserie chicken) is their specialty along with a zillion different fish and over 3,000 varieties of potato. Consequently, my wife orders chicken or fish at every restaurant and her heart breaks if they don't bring the head on the fish. The point is that her entire country, and much of South America, has this principle down to the letter. It is a natural way of life and it helps their citizens default to the healthy choice. Everyone else can too. It's just a matter of training yourself and building menu-ordering habits. Believe me, it won't take long for you to feel the health benefits of it. You will not feel as bloated and tired. You will sleep better and have more energy. Our bodies don't need pills and powders for energy and health. They need fresh F&V/F&C.

SWEETS

People love to say, "I can't give up my sweets." Well, every sweet is not created equal. Sorbet is super sweet. Berries with Cool Whip® is super sweet and so is double chocolate cake. It's time you get a grip on your sweet tooth. If sweet is really your need, then you can get it 1,000 different ways. But if you are trying to justify a slab of chocolate cheesecake, then good luck reaching your health goals. It's as simple as that. Eat all the cookies you want, but don't turn around and wonder why you are not losing weight, improving your numbers or feeling better. Remember, too, we are not *sacrificing*, we are *substituting*. It is completely fine to have your sweets. Just redefine them or keep the less healthy ones to a minimum.

By the way, I can't leave this subject without mentioning the fact that I launched a campaign called *Fsugar.org*. This is a challenge to give up anything with sugar on its label for twenty-four hours. (Fruits and vegetables don't have labels, so they are okay.) Believe me, it is not easy. The challenge is primarily to get people to focus on the sugar content in everything they consume, from milk to mayonnaise. One of the most brainless things you can do is simply look at the sugar content on the label affixed to virtually every single packaged or processed thing you eat. In the past, people looked at calories. Then they started fixating on fat. These days they look at carbs (which turn into sugar if not burned), but sugar is a really simple thing to keep an eye on. Food labels are useful, and if you only look at one thing, look at *the sugar.*

You will be absolutely blown away when you flip over a fruit juice and discover that it has 58 grams of sugar. That's 20 grams *more* than a Coke. If that brainless behavior doesn't get you to start reconsidering your choices, you have bigger problems to solve.

There is no amount of exercise that will combat that kind of sugar assault. The World Health Organization (WHO) states that men should have no more than 35 grams of sugar and women should have no more than 25 grams a day. I hope you are sitting down, because the *average American ingests 180 grams of sugar every single day*. No wonder that more than 100 million Americans either have diabetes or prediabetes. That's over one in three American adults. If you can't cut that number down in your diet, then it really doesn't matter what you do with the rest of your life. You are going to suffer. Your body just can't handle that kind of sugar onslaught.

By now it should be clear that sugar can be deadly. Just ask anyone with a relative that has died of diabetes or suffers every day with the disease. At the levels that most people eat sugar, they might as well suck up arsenic through a straw. It will crash the natural insulin pump in your pancreas and create a condition called *insulin resistance*, which ushers in diabetes. On top of that organ-destroying effect, excess sugar turns into fat, which leads to obesity. In 2013, obesity was designated as a chronic *disease* by the American Medical Society because it is linked to heart disease, Alzheimer's and cancer *in addition* to diabetes, stroke and kidney failure.

My work with the CDC has included almost a decade of projects involving the National Diabetes Prevention Program, known as the National DPP. This evidence-based program is proven to reverse the condition of prediabetes and prevent diabetes. Plus, it is nearly twice as effective as the leading diabetes medications.

No cost for medicine, no side effects from medicine and no deadly disease. Sounds pretty brainless to me. You can find out if you happen to be the one in three Americans who currently has prediabetes by going to *DoIHavePrediabetes.org* and taking a one-minute risk test. If your risk-score is high enough, you may qualify to enroll in the National DPP. You can learn more at *www.cdc.gov/prediabetes*. Ask your employer or insurance company if it covers it. DPP costs less than a set of tires for your car and far less than a new iPhone, but hey, if you can get it paid for, then go for it. Regardless, check out your risk for prediabetes pronto. It's not something to mess around with.

Here's another relatively brainless tip when it comes to eating with other people, whether at home or at a restaurant: focus on the *people* you are with and not the food. Focus on the conversation and the time together and let food be secondary. Too often, food is our drug. Food is the main event. Food is the thing we focus on and the thing that satisfies. In fact, if the food is bad, we are not just upset with the meal, but upset with the evening and upset with the moment. Conversely, if we can view our friends as the entrée, then you will rarely be disappointed.

I know, you are probably saying, "You are crazy; food *is* the *fun*. It *is* the main event whether we go out or stay in." I hear you. I'm just saying that when you reduce food to a form of sustenance, instead of an emotional orgasm, then you are going to be better equipped to order the healthy options.

Remember, healthy habits will always involve some level of discipline at the beginning. Then they magically transform into being brainless. Your diet is no different.

CONVICTION

On the heels of discipline and consistency must come *conviction*. I think it is amazing how relatively easy it seems for most vegetarians, vegans or pescatarians to be disciplined about their food choices.

I have interviewed many such people, and while I discovered that their initial behavioral change certainly required discipline, what made them maintain was their conviction. They were motivated by something higher, such as religion, or morality toward animals or a belief about the dangers of certain foods. As a result, I have never heard any of my vegan/vegetarian/pescatarian friends whine about not being able to have a juicy steak. Rather, it is an anathema to them. It is not even a temptation. Conversely, when someone becomes a vegan/vegetarian/pescatarian *without* that higher conviction, it rarely sticks. Cultural fads don't motivate like conviction.

The lesson to learn is to develop a higher consciousness toward *your* healthy habits. Discipline will play a critical role to *establish* the habit, but conviction will *sustain* it. Perhaps you will learn about the damaging effects of too much sugar on your endocrine system and suddenly you will begin to view a cupcake with six inches of icing as something you'd rather avoid in lieu of something less sugary. Perhaps you will learn about the antioxidant properties of certain vegetables and you will suddenly start adding a salad to your meal without even thinking about it because you want those nutrients in your body on a regular basis. It just becomes a habit based on a heart-felt conviction. Soon, the temptation abates, and the struggle dissipates. Try it and see.

When it comes to starting your new disciplines around food, let me introduce you to a few fresh ideas (besides portion control, etc.) that helped me change my behavior.

THEY WON'T STOP MAKING YUMMY FOOD

That is so brainless we tend to forget it. Recently I was at a movie with a friend and he said that he wanted popcorn. I told him to go ahead and get it. Then I added, "Or you can have it the next time you go to the movies." He wasn't going to stop going to the movies, and there will always be piles of fake-buttery popcorn waiting for him there. Same with those potato chips at the grocery store or that candy bar at the gas station. Don't view discipline as something you have to give up *forever*. Don't even tell yourself to cut back. Just remind yourself that you can have it *later*. Then when later comes, you will realize that you survived without it and it will dawn on you that maybe you can survive without it again.

I did that with pizza, which used to rule my life. Pizza is my all-time favorite food. I love the taste, the smell, the heat and even the anticipation of it. I used to order pizza any time just for the fun of it. It was that much of a drug to me. It was also a coping mechanism when things were not going well. Then one day, I told myself, *I will just order it tomorrow.* When tomorrow came, I was traveling, or we already had dinner plans, or it was too late. Bottom line, I lived another day without pizza, and I didn't shrivel up and die. I didn't even care. That is the point. I taught myself that I really could live without something that I thought I couldn't. Putting it off was different than forbidding myself from eating it. It is simple. It is brainless. It works.

OCCASIONALLY INDULGE

One of the reasons we love vacations is that we don't have them every day. Same with Christmas and Thanksgiving. We don't eat a massive stuffed turkey every day, or pumpkin pie. These are things that we look forward to just like seasonal Starbucks drinks. I love every single drop of the 380 calories in a tall pumpkin spiced latte as a seasonal ritual. I don't mind indulging because it's special. Of course, I could drink one every day for three months, but I don't because it would become routine or even boring. Maximize your pleasure by making indulging special.

I have always hated the concept of a *cheat day.* That's a day when those on a diet get to eat anything they want. First, that flies in the face of developing sustainable eating habits and a healthy daily diet that does not include restricting or depriving yourself. Second, I don't like the term *cheat.* I'm not a prude, but since when was cheating a good thing in *any* context, and who exactly are we cheating if it is *our* diet? The answer is *ourselves.* We lose out when we scarf down that pint of ice cream or box of cookies. Cheaters always cheat themselves. So, if you must indulge, then go ahead and indulge, but call it *a treat day*, **not a cheat day**.

BUY NOW, EAT LATER

A while ago, I bought a massive bag of M&Ms. Actually, I bought two. We are talking the biggest bag that the Mars company manufactures. I did it because they are my favorite candy and they were on a massive after-Christmas sale. What could be better? They were just the red and green ones, and I checked the expiration date to discover that I could enjoy cost savings for my sweet cravings for the next nine months. Having things on hand can be very dangerous, but it can also be strategic. That's because when I am tempted to order dessert at a restaurant, I remember that I have a whole bag of M&Ms waiting for me at home, and because I love them so much I am able to forego the purchase of dessert. Typically, by the time I get home I have forgotten all about my sweet tooth. It's brainless.

Purchasing things for later consumption alleviates both the feeling of deprivation and the relative panic I have about not being able to find some sweets later. Sure, I just said that the yummy food manufacturers will keep making yummy food, but in the case of my after-Christmas candy bonanza, I got caught thinking that I wouldn't find them *on sale* later, so I just bought them. It worked. I got them, and I stored them. No problem. Chill out and purchase. Don't feel guilty or indulgent. Chances are you will end up throwing half of them out after they expire.

Sadly, I never ate a single M&M out of either of those massive bags because even though they were completely sealed, they somehow attracted ants to the cabinet where I had hidden them. My wife discovered the ants, and to purge the infestation she threw out both bags. There you have it. Temptation gone.

While still on the subject of sweets, let me introduce you to what I call the *One Bite Appetite*.

No one wants to live in a world without desserts. I certainly don't. I love desserts. But typically, I love the *taste* of the sweetness. At the risk of introducing too much science, researchers at Boston University School of Management and the Stanford University Graduate School of Business replicated previous findings on *sensory-specific satiety*. That means that each bite of food is less pleasant than the one before it. (See: https://www.psychologicalscience.org/news/releases/its-the-last-bite-that-keeps-you-coming-back-for-more.html.)

Our taste buds light up at the *first taste* of something. That's why we want to eat a second bite. So, I typically have a *single bite* of dessert. Or, I have one bite of *someone else's* dessert. (It costs a lot less). Sometimes, I break off just one piece of a chocolate bar, which is all I need to satisfy my sweet tooth. Sure, I *could* eat the whole thing. Sure, I *want* to eat the whole thing. But typically, I remember this rule of one bite, and to this day it's always satisfied me.

If you stick to the *One Bite Appetite* principle, you can theoretically have dessert at every single meal. Seriously, think about it. That's just three bites a day. It won't even add up to one single full dessert. It's brainless. The same goes for single servings of mashed potatoes, stuffing, and other high- or bad-calorie indulgences. Just eat what's on your plate and wipe your mouth. It's what we do in restaurants. We don't order a second entrée, so don't return for seconds in your home.

PEER PRESSURES

Peer pressure is as toxic for adults as it is for teenagers. People want you to order the onion rings when they are doing so. They love for you to order dessert when they are, and they certainly want you to have an alcoholic drink with them. They will say, "Go for it" and will tell you that you look great and you don't need to diet. In fact, they will shame you for dieting. They wouldn't even understand if you told them that you are *not on a diet*, but that your regular eating habits are part of your regular diet. It's super hard. One solution is to hang out with other healthy people. Get some positive peer pressure for a change. If you apply the brainless principle of surrounding yourself with healthy people, then it's likely that the negative peer pressure around food will vanish.

Case in point: I recently ran a 5K with 1,000 people who showed up on a hot summer Saturday at 7:30 in the morning. They were all shapes and sizes and ages, but they all had health in common. These people were universally committed to living a healthy life. I absolutely love fitness events like 5Ks because they are the entry point for what I call *the other public health, the kind of health that you demonstrate in public.* That's big. When you slip into your spandex in front of the general public, you mean business.

Even at marathons and triathlons, you will discover that competitors are still wildly accepting, encouraging and represent all skill levels. When I did my first (and only) triathlon, I was super scared. I was sure I might drown in the swim. I envisioned people kicking me in the head as I gasped for air. I was sure I would crumple during the final run. Instead, I finished strong and without embarrassing myself. I didn't get a flat tire. I didn't puke during the run. And I didn't drown. Part of the reason was because everyone was cheering each other on. It was nuts. My actual competitors were cheering me on as I passed them. Plus, there were fans along the race route cheering me on. These were people who just loved the racing community who had come out to cheer for health.

When you are surrounded by such positivity, you emulate it. You want to fuel that fire. You want to make them proud, so to speak. You want to be like them. Believe me, it's bizarre. I've never seen anything like it and I sure love it.

I encourage everyone to enter a 5K, 10K, half marathon, etc. just to check out the people. They are not all Olympians. Far from it. But they are all committed to health. They are the type that have fun, drink beer and eat pizza on occasion, but they don't make a habit of crushing a twelve-pack of beer and a bag of Doritos. They are the kinds of friends you want alongside you. They will absolutely destroy any negative peer pressure in your life and improve every aspect of your life far beyond physical health.

Speaking of which, it's time we turn our attention to emotional and mental health that impacts your physical health 100 percent of the time.

CHAPTER SEVENTEEN

CONNECTION PROTECTION

SCIENCE HAS FOUND that loneliness is downright deadly. Visit https://artandhealing.org and you will discover on the home page of the *Unlonely Project* a startling fact that "loneliness is as lethal as smoking fifteen cigarettes a day." Read that again. *Fifteen cigarettes.* No toxic chemicals and no nicotine, but plenty of toxic combustion going on, *inside* your body and literally attacking your organs.

Studies reveal that negative emotions can have horrible physiological effects on your body. According to the American Academy of Family Physicians, negative emotions can cause high blood pressure, stomach ulcers, compromised immune system (leading to sickness and infection), constipation, and insomnia. The complete list is long and disturbing. That's not counting clinical depression or other diagnosable mental illnesses. The University of Minnesota goes so far as to say that negative attitudes can create chronic stress, which upsets the body's hormone balance, depletes the brain chemicals, damages the immune system and actually decreases our lifespan by shortening our telomeres (the "end caps" of our DNA strands), which *causes us to age more quickly.* You not only die sooner, but you are going to look worse in your casket.

The project states, "For many people, loneliness is not simply an occasional feeling, but a corrosive burden on their health, well-being, and sense of self." *Corrosive.* That is a powerful word. Loneliness is also known as *social isolation.* It is not simply a feeling, but a state of being in your own world, be it your place of employment, your neighborhood, or even your family. You either are physically isolated, such as shut inside your home, or you simply *feel* isolated. The *feeling* of isolation is far more rampant than most people realize. Sometimes it is hard for the person suffering from isolation to recognize it because they are constantly surrounded by people they don't acknowledge.

Many traveling salespeople report being lonely. People in sales are typically extroverted and always around others, but inside they can be lonely. They travel alone, stay in hotels alone, eat alone and feel detached from meaningful relationships. One of my closest friends is uber-connected to movers and shakers, societal networks and country club backslappers, but admits to being alone. He only has a few close friends and most of them are too busy to connect. Remember that time is what counts. Not people on your LinkedIn account. Not friends on Facebook. Those people are not accessible in times of need, or more importantly, in times *before* need. We need relational connection before the proverbial shit hits the fan.

I remember ten years ago when I was in crisis and I called my three best friends. Within twenty-four hours they were all at my door. Dan from Kansas, Jimmy from Maryland and Scott from Georgia. It wasn't simply because I was in crisis. It was because I was their friend and I had nurtured and pruned and cared for those relationships *before* I had the ultimate need for those relationships.

Relationships take time and maintenance. They must be mutually beneficial and fertilized like a tree or plant, which is difficult in our culture. We are busy people, and yet we have to recognize that it is essential to our overall health and theirs. We must add relationships to our to-do list. They don't come naturally.

I suggest selecting three or four people that you really like and then brainlessly reaching out to them every week. It doesn't have to be deep. Send them a picture when you are out. Tell them you wish they were there. Give them some insight into your life. It's so incredibly easy today to send a text, shoot a picture, drop an email, forward an Instagram or Facetime them these days. In the past, you needed to stay tethered to your kitchen phone for a chat or pen a letter, and, heaven forbid, find a stamp. If you really want to blow someone away, invest the time it takes to write a letter. Go for it. They will be floored. It will deliver an added level of value to their life. People don't do this anymore, and therefore it will elevate your friendship. It will accentuate your commitment to them. People who take the time to write a letter are people who are worth investing in.

While we are on the topic of relationships, let's not forget family. What if you took the time to write a letter to a family member? We often take our family for granted, yet they can be some of the sweetest friends if we treat them right and nurture those relationships. I remember calling my sisters almost every day during one of my darkest times. After that, I let it go. The storms passed, and I got busy again. Not cool. So, I started reaching out again. How many people do you know who are no longer close with the people they grew up with? Tons. It is rare to find siblings and grandparents and uncles who stay close till the end. What a lost opportunity. What a lost precious resource. These people *often* know us best. No matter how much we think we have changed, these are the people we grew up with. These are the people who care about us the most. At the end of the day, blood really is thicker than water, and often these are the easiest relationships to maintain but also the easiest to ignore. We must nurture these relationships.

We've all seen the movie scenes that show some lonely character sitting at the bar pouring his/her heart out to the bartender or a perfect stranger. That is not just a Hollywood cliché; that is reflective of our society, and it is not healthy.

Today, loneliness affects 30 percent of Americans. AARP conducted a study that found that loneliness has *doubled* since 1980. That should seem both surprising and not surprising at the same time. One would think that our social media and mobile devices would keep us connected and engaged, but alas it creates a special, new barrier. Today it is not uncommon for people to text each other in the same house, room to room.

Often, we might choose to text happy birthday greetings to avoid having to speak with someone and cover more topics than the actual birthday. Our social media tools are a way of checking the box of social interaction without having to engage in any actual social interaction. The next time you text or email or post, stop in the middle of it and look around. You are most likely alone. You are isolated. Then hit send or finish your post. Now look around. You are still alone, and you have figuratively hung up the phone with your friend. You have disconnected. You have disengaged, and likely you are on to another social post or off to do some other activity. At the end of the day, all the posts and texts in the world do not stimulate the brain the same way as a face-to-face or voice-to-voice conversation. They can be powerful, but not in the same way. You do not receive the same feelings of connectedness.

I'm not saying that social media or digital communications is bad. I still get plenty of emotions when my wife flirts with me via text. I love it. Studies have shown that people express similar facial reactions reading a digital message as those in face-to-face interactions. Our hearts can still flutter just seeing the bubbles of a text being composed from a lover or loved one.

The bottom line is that however you relate, relationships are key to preventing damaging health effects. Even if you are not around your closest friends very often, just knowing that they are a phone call away can stave off loneliness and medicate your physical being.

A 2015 review of over thirty years of research found that loneliness also has the same health risks of obesity, with loneliness increasing the likelihood of death by up to 32 percent, according to research by J. Holt-Lunstad, T. Smith, M. Baker, T. Harris, & D. Stephenson. (2015). I'm not making this stuff up. Get back to being brainless and reach out to your friends. Get connected. This is not rocket science. This is not as hard as going to the gym or eating healthy. This has historically been a natural behavior, and if it has become unnatural for you, it is time to self-examine.

The Loneliness Project's website also discusses the five areas of loneliness connected to family, friends, romantic partners, self and spirituality. (See: www.lonelinessproject.org)

WORK AND LONELINESS

When it comes to work, most employees are quick to embrace tele-work if given the option. Today, according to GlobalWorkplaceAnalytics.com, up to 25 percent of full-time employees tele-work, but 80 to 90 percent wish they could. This is fascinating. Of course, everyone thinks of the upside, the ability to log on to the company intranet while sipping a cup of coffee in their pajamas. They can throw a load of laundry in the dryer while they wait to join the conference call. They can water the plants, do the dishes or prep dinner all while answering emails and drafting the latest PowerPoint. It is great. But over time, it leads to isolation. Even if kids are running around the house, it isn't the same as adult interaction. It is not the same as collegial conversation and the respect and confidence that can come with it. Not dressing for success at work can also take its toll on our psychological and emotional and professional health, to say nothing of our intimate relationships. If sweatpants become your typical work-week attire, don't forget that someone else in your family might be coming home and hoping to see you in something more attractive. According to Chron.com, "staff who communicate only online and by phone may have a harder time retaining and building relationships with their colleagues, which can sabotage overall productivity and job satisfaction. Because relationships often lead to trust and effective collaboration, telecommuting can weaken the overall atmosphere."

I tele-work and I love it, but it diminishes the overall connectedness I feel toward my colleagues. When I got married, there was a dissipated sharing of my big event with my close colleagues simply because I wasn't around. That can result in real detachment. A colleague recently told me she had separated from her husband. I was dumbstruck and asked her when it happened, assuming it must have been just weeks ago. She said that it happened six months earlier. I was floored. That's how out of touch I was simply due to our new tele-work policy.

The website *Launch Worksites* contends that face-to-face interactions at work (as opposed to tele-work) have the following benefits.

Builds trust and credibility

Meeting in person allows you to show your true personality, emotions, and reactions. It helps you build a more meaningful connection with potential partners and clients, helps build credibility and establishes trust and loyalty. Relationships grow best through face-to-face interaction. You know this to be true.

Increases productivity

A twenty-five-message email thread could be boiled down to five minutes of in-person speaking if people would just pick up the phone. Tasks are accomplished quicker, and misinterpretation and misunderstanding are minimized. Face-to-face communication also boosts collaboration and creativity through the ability to share ideas more freely.

Allows you to read nonverbal cues

Communication is more than just words. Conversing with people in person helps you detect body language, feelings, tone, and reactions, which can *often* be misinterpreted through digital means.

The idea in bullet point number one is paramount. The idea of building relationships and especially earning trust via face-to-face interaction cannot be overstated. When was the last time you built a relationship (from ground zero) via text? Online dating is legend. You show up and the person is not like their picture or even the conversations that you had via email and text.

Regardless of whether you tele-work or report to an office, when it comes to work relationships, it's hard to be brainless. Work is generally complex, political, difficult, stressful and full of multiple personality types. It is hard enough to navigate with your brain fully engaged, let alone running in the background of your life. Therefore, I don't want you to overthink this other than to begin to value your work relationships—even the difficult ones—and build them in person when at all possible.

I used to have a tough relationship with one of my colleagues at work for seven years, but I worked on it every day. I valued it and I used it to gauge the growth of my professionalism. Every now and then, this colleague would compliment or thank me, and it did wonders for my ego. It meant more than all the praise from the other colleagues with whom I had a great relationship. It brought health to my psyche. It made me feel like I was growing and improving and maturing. It made me feel better about myself and my professional progress.

RELATIONAL LONELINESS

Now, let's get really personal and talk about *personal* relationships, again. I've already touched on this regarding intimacy, but personal relationships are much broader. They are the ultimate source of feeling connected to this world and to a purpose larger than ourselves. They also directly contribute to feelings of health and wellbeing, or they can cause significant levels of stress and anguish.

This isn't a guide to marital counseling, conflict resolution or a primer on how to win friends and influence people, but I want you to stop and reflect on how your most important relationships directly impact your health. Think of a love that you won or lost. You can probably recall the emotion with just one thought. Think of how that impacted other areas of your life. Think about your best friend or the one that betrayed you. Think about the hole that it left in your life. Think about someone who passed away and the ache it caused you.

Connecting relationship health with physical health is just logical. Emotions can give us the sweats or increase our heartrate or shorten our breath. Each is a physical reaction. Personal relationships can cause our palms to become damp or clammy. Conversely, relationships can also cause us to relax or give us a sense of security or deep peace. Our heart rate can slow. Our skin can warm. Our eyes might brighten. Sometimes we even start to salivate. All these physical reactions are directly connected to our emotional state.

As I have already stated, friendships have a uniquely powerful impact on our health. That is because friends are people who *choose* to spend time with you, *choose* to call you, *choose* to share their lives with you, *choose* to love you. They are different than even the best family members because of the choice they make, repeatedly, to be with you. They chose you. Similarly, there is great power in knowing that you are choosing to be with others. Our gift of friendship *to others* can be as life giving as a ventilator or pacemaker.

Sometimes, the closest relationships in our life can inspire us to greatness. They can give us the support we need to try new things and take new risks. Specific to our health, our relationships can motivate us to embrace healthy lifestyle behaviors that allow us to live long enough to *love and be loved by those we love.* Typically, people have many different reasons for hanging around this planet. The goal is to get in touch with your own personal reason, focus on that reason, and then take steps to make sure you achieve it while helping those around you achieve their own goals.

A colleague of mine wrote down her reason to exercise on an index card and laminated it. She carries it in her computer case so that she will see it every day. It simply says, "You want to be an active grandmother." That's it. Her relationship with her grandson is her greatest motivation to care for her own health.

Children and grandchildren can provide massive motivation for connection. Kids have probably been more responsible for getting their parents to quit smoking than any other reason. They pester them relentlessly (as only kids can do) and have been known to throw their parents' cigarettes in the trash or down the toilet.

Unfortunately, immediate familial relationships can sometimes be so time consuming that we fail to develop and maintain close non-family friendships. In today's frenetic, overscheduled and fast-paced world, it is easy for friendships and *familyships* to fall into the optional category, like vacations and adequate sleep. We simply view friendships as a luxury that we can't afford or don't deserve. I cannot begin to count the number of times friends have told me they are too busy to go out or too tired to meet up or too overextended to attend a party. That's insane. That is not healthy living. That's not fun living.

The truth is that friendships should not be an option. We cannot afford to *not* invest in friends. When we were kids, making friends was brainless. We didn't consider whether to make them or not, we just did it. We ran onto the playground and made friends, instantly. That's the brainlessness to which we must return as busy adults.

Recently, we moved into a new neighborhood. Job one was making cookies for our neighbors. We *automatically* (brainlessly) decided that we would not wait around for someone to knock on our door with a fresh-made pie. Rather, we would raise the flag of friendship ourselves. It wasn't even a question. We didn't debate it or spy on our neighbors to see if they seemed worthy of the effort. We just baked the cookies and delivered them. That's brainless friendship. That's brainless community. That's brainless health.

LOVE RELATIONSHIPS

I love this topic because it's so completely straightforward.

I believe that a lot of couples' therapists would go out of business if lovers were able to remember what they were thinking when they fell in love. Despite what we like to believe, to justify our drama, romantic relationships are not rocket science. Most involve attraction, infatuation, electricity, and tenderness. At least that's how they start and, predictably, if those things disappear, the relationship will start to suck. Therefore, *don't let that happen.*

See? Pretty simple. But of course, it's *not* easy. Fortunately, it is very achievable if we are willing to create automatic, brainless behaviors that run in the background of our relationship. What's not so simple is harnessing our tendencies toward jealousy, impatience, laziness, selfishness, and our ever-demanding ego. So, the goal is to maintain those early sparks, fan them into flames from time to time and make sure the fire never goes out completely. The ways to do that are varied and creative but they are not secrets. Nothing is a secret now that the internet exits. Just Google *how to add romance to my marriage* or *how to keep my relationship alive* or *how to keep humping after you've been humping a long time.* Below are my own top five super brainless relationship pointers:

1. **Stay attractive to the other person**. You may not have been a fitness model or wearing Italian leather when you met, but you were physically and emotionally attractive to your lover in some way. Don't stray from those days. Take care of your body and your wardrobe. Don't devolve into slovenly

dress just because you see each other with bedhead and bad breath. Step up your physical attractiveness game at every opportunity. Few people fall in love with a slob, but many find themselves married to one just a few years later. Aim to maintain the person you were. Better yet, *try* to improve yourself. Get in better shape, dress better, improve your style. Be that person again. Be that person every day.

2. **Stay kind and polite**. Don't complain about the other person or tell them what to do or make them feel little or stupid or dismissed. Don't create expectations of the other person. You used to do your own laundry, so why expect someone else to do it now? Learn to cook or clean. Share the load. Lend a hand. Open the door. Say I'm sorry. Say I love you. Say I appreciate you. Follow the Golden Rule. You know what *you* want, so do *that*.

3. **Keep surprising**. Keep giving gifts, planning dates, going on trips or even just making dinner. If doing the laundry would be a surprise to your lover, then do that. Drop notes in the mail, leave them under the pillow. Pick up flowers at the grocery, or at the gas station. Just do it and do it and do it again.

4. **Truly listen**. Stop and care enough to listen about their day or their dreams. Do it authentically. Listening involves remembering what someone told you later. It is an active activity. Remove distractions and pay attention when you ask a question. People can tell when you aren't listening. Don't ask a question if you are not able to focus on the answer. Someone once said, "We have two ears and one mouth, so we need to listen twice as much as we talk." Brainless.

5. **Serve each other.** Help each other with easy things and hard things. Take out the trash, clean up the dishes, make the bed, hang the picture, iron the clothes, turn off the lights, cancel

the cable, order the part, mail the package, make the bed. You get it. Take time to do it.

The bottom line is, like most things, you *already know what to do*. It's stuff you did when you fell in love. Just keep doing those things. Don't let routine or stress or change win the war. Try to outdo the other person in those five areas and you will wildly increase your chances of staying in love.

NON-HUMAN RELATIONSHIPS

While a lot of people love animals, there is a growing number of people who love them more than humans. Regardless of your affinity for animals or people, having a pet is healthy. Coming home to a dog that jumps on you and greets you like you are the best human on planet Earth makes you feel good. It makes you feel needed. It ruins your clothes, but you don't care. Your emotions get a healthy boost.

When it comes to dogs, there are practical physical benefits. You have to walk it (or at least you have the option to walk it) which ends up taking *you* on a walk. You have to get up and down to feed it, groom it or simply open the back door or get out of bed when it barks. It's like having a two-year-old who never grows up. Basically, it keeps you moving. Even cats, while far less demanding, provide immeasurable company, affection and unconditional love. They also require us to serve someone other than ourselves.

Pets can also have a calming, anti-stress effect. One of my colleagues deals with an inordinate amount of stress at his job. Recently we went to a meeting and in trotted a dog. Instantly, my colleague started petting the dog. He later told me that simply *seeing the dog* and being in its presence during the meeting reduced his stress level significantly. It was my first experience having a pet in a business setting, but the effect on my colleague improved the meeting immensely. Since that day, I've advocated for pets in our office, imagining the wonders it could do for other stressed-out employees.

I have personally had many pets over the years and most recently we brought home a hamster. I did not want the hamster. I did not want to feed it, change its cage, or listen to its wheel all night.

Nevertheless, after a few months I found myself talking to the fur ball. If I was working late at night, downstairs alone, I'd pick her up and talk to her. I'd say goodbye to her before I left the house, and I'd greet her upon my return. I monitored every aspect of her living conditions. It was bizarre to me, but completely in line with the research about humans and their pets.

If you don't have a pet and are entertaining getting one, I suggest a hamster because they are cheap to buy and keep. They are also easy to pawn off to a friend when you travel, and you never need to cut your dinner date short because you have to get home to let the hamster out. Sure, there are limitations. You can't exactly wrestle with a hamster or take them for a walk, but if you are considering pet ownership for the first time, it's a safe place to start.

REACH OUT AND TOUCH

Today, most of us live in a rather touch-free world. Just like those touch-free car washes that blast the dirt off without any slippery chamois ever touching your car's paint, so our society is strung together by smart phones, email and mobile apps that never require us to touch another human being. Science tells us that touch is a very basic human need and we should give it and seek it, regularly.

Many studies show that babies deprived of physical touch end up being at greater risk of social, emotional and physical problems later in life. According to Dr. Frank Lipman, author of the book *How to Be Well*, when you are touched in a meaningful way, such as a warm hug, your body releases tension, stress levels go down and your immune system actually gets a boost. It seems crazy, but it's not. Lipman even gets into the science. He believes that hugs trigger the vagus nerve, which relaxes you and also tells your brain to release oxytocin, which boosts self-esteem and reduces anxiety and feelings of aloneness.

When I entered the field of public health, I had no idea how much hugging would be involved. Most people in the field are women, and women know how to nurture and touch and hug. Add to that the fact that most people are in public health because they are committed to helping people. Therefore, hugging is kind of a natural extension of their work. It was bizarrely uncomfortable for me at first, but now I find it both normal and desirable. In fact, I recently said goodbye to a colleague at the airport and as we rushed to our planes we didn't have time to hug. I caught myself missing that collegial, physical connection.

I have read stories of marriages that were at the brink of divorce and were turned around simply by reintroducing touch. A simple handhold. A simple kiss to the forehead. It isn't magic; it is the way we are wired, and it works. You know it to be true. You know that you love to touch and be touched at least by the ones you love. So, do it. Get it. Give it and build it into the way you live and breathe. Even a handshake is touch. So, get touching. Your health will thank you. It's brainless.

CHAPTER EIGHTEEN

GET VERTICAL

JUST LIKE LONELINESS, THE negative health effects of being sedentary are associated with smoking. In fact, sitting has been called the *new smoking*. That's how damaging it is to your health.

When was the last time you *fell asleep* standing? However, it is extremely common to fall asleep on the couch, in an airplane seat, on a train, or at our desk. That's because sitting puts the body to sleep. It's as simple as that and that is what you must remember. That's the brainless tip: stand periodically, even while watching a TV show or typing an email, and you will force your body to work, burn calories, and increase oxygen.

Welcome to the standing desk revolution.

I don't know exactly when standing desks came into vogue, but they are here to stay. The fact is that standing desks are in every modern office today and no one looks at you strangely if you have one. I'm no trend setter or futurist, but I am observant, and twenty years ago I discovered that I was more productive standing than sitting. I simply jacked up my desk on a set of milk crates (stylish, I know) and my first standing desk was born. I discovered that I didn't take as much time deliberating over linguistical nuances in my emails. I just hammered them out because I removed the ability to lean back in my cushy chair, scratch my scruffy chin and ponder the English language.

Years later, I had a desk that precluded the use of milk crates, so I simply grabbed a file box and placed it on top of my desk and then put my laptop computer on top of it. *Voile!* I had my second standing desk. Finally, last year our company sprang for a legitimate, factory-made standing desk, and I've never been happier at the office. It is empowering. It gives me a psychological edge. I feel in charge. I feel like I'm at the helm of a ship. It's my make-believe lectern. It's my Starfleet command center.

It makes me more productive and seems to allow me to think clearer. According to Teeter.com, standing desks have real health benefits. They cite:

Reduced back pain. In 2011, they launched a "Take-a-Stand Project" and found that participants who spent an average of sixty-six minutes of their workday standing experienced a 54 percent reduction in upper back and neck pain.

Reduced risk of heart disease. Researchers have been studying the benefits of standing for more than sixty years. In 1953 a study of bus conductors found that those who stood all day had half the risk of heart disease–related deaths compared to the bus drivers who were seated. https://www.ncbi.nlm.nih.gov/pmc/articles/PMC2027542/

Reduced risk of weight gain and obesity. By standing instead of sitting, you can reduce the risk of weight gain by burning approximately fifty extra calories an hour. If you were to stand for three hours each workday, it would be equal to 750 calories a week. Over the course of a full year that would equal about 30,000 extra calories burned, or about eight pounds of fat. In terms of activity levels, those 30,000 calories would be the equivalent of running ten marathons a year. https://www.ncbi.nlm.nih.gov/pubmed/24297826

Reduced risk of type 2 diabetes. In 2013, a small study of ten office workers showed that standing for 180 minutes after lunch reduced the workers' blood sugar levels by 43 percent compared to sitting for the same time period. https://www.ncbi.nlm.nih.gov/pubmed/24297826

Another study of twenty-three overweight office workers found that alternating every thirty minutes between standing and sitting reduced blood sugar spikes by an average of 11.1 percent. https://www.ncbi.nlm.nih.gov/pubmed/24637345

Improved mood and energy. During the "Take-a-Stand Project" in 2011, a group of twenty-four office workers were provided with a standing desk. Participants self-reported *an improvement in their mood* over the four weeks where they reduced their time sitting by an average of sixty-six minutes. https://www.ncbi.nlm.nih.gov/pubmed/23057991

At the end of the four-week intervention period, participants were asked a series of questions regarding the specific benefits of alternating between sitting and standing positions. The results: 87 percent felt more comfortable; 87 percent felt energized; 75 percent felt healthier; 71 percent felt more focused; 66 percent felt more productive; 62 percent felt happier; 33 percent felt less stressed as a result of having the standing workstations. When the sit-stand desks were removed, the participants reported a deterioration in mood.

BOOST PRODUCTIVITY

The boost in mood and energy, as well as the reduction in back, shoulder, and neck pain, is likely to improve productivity and mental alertness. When the body as a whole is in better shape, it functions more efficiently, and it can be reasonably expected that this would in turn boost productivity.

I have a friend who preaches *movement after meals*. This brainless concept simply involves standing from the table and moving, *in some way*, after your meal. It doesn't matter if you walk the dog or walk around your home or office—just move. Allow the blood to circulate and the heart to pump to aid in digestion. Don't get up from the breakfast table and simply sit down again in your car and drive to the office. Go get the mail. Walk around the backyard. Take the stairs up to your bedroom. Similarly, don't finish dinner and get in bed or sit on the couch. Move one way or another and help your body with its digestion, metabolism, and blood flow. It's brainless. *Eat, drink, move.*

A few years ago, the National Association of Chronic Disease Directors spearheaded a movement simply called *Get Vertical*. The idea was simply to stand and do anything that would allow the blood to flow. The idea of standing or straightening the body is so simple but so easily forgotten. After all, sitting feels good. Sitting is relaxing. Sitting is comfortable. Sitting is programmed into our environment.

I love step-tracking devices that tell you when it is time to stand. Recently, my colleague was driving a group of us to a business meeting three hours away across Alaska. He told us that he would be pulling the car over on the road in order to stand, whenever his watch prompted him to do so. He received points for achieving his prescribed number of standing goals each day and he wasn't going to miss out on his point accumulation just because he was on a road trip. It may have been extreme, but no one cared, and everyone in the car got a chance to stretch their legs when we pulled over. Like I said at the beginning of the book, it's the twenty-first century and health is hip. Health is cool. Take a stand. Health is the new black!

CHAPTER NINETEEN

MINDFUL HYGIENE

MOST PARENTS SPEND a good part of their life trying to teach their children personal hygiene. They know that it will serve them in a million ways from their health to their relationships to their careers. But believe me, today's personal hygiene goes way beyond clipping your toenails.

There's no other part of this book that has such unanimous support, yet few people know just how many illnesses can be avoided by practicing *mindful* hygiene.

The Australian government's Department of Health lists poor personal hygiene as a *leading cause* of human hookworms, threadworms, roundworms and pinworms in your anus. Nice, huh? Avoiding bodily parasites should be among everyone's top ten life objectives.

In addition to being contracted from other unhygienic persons, head lice can originate from lack of good personal hygiene. By the way, if you have ever had lice personally or had it in your family, you know that it is a nightmare to eliminate and will cause you to boil every stitch of clothing and every bed sheet that you have. Washing your clothes and sheets regularly can greatly reduce the chance of nasty diseases.

Similarly, many foodborne illnesses that will cause you to vomit up your lungs, if they don't kill you, can arrive simply from leaving food out or not storing it well. So, clean up your space as well as your body.

Emptying trash regularly—completely—is key. Wiping toilet seats and scrubbing out your toilet (yep, that's what those brushes are for) is also critical. Human feces is prime for transmitting disease. If I didn't make it painfully clear enough earlier, washing your hands is the single most brainless thing you can do. It's downright fundamental to controlling the transmission of germs to your nose when you decide to pick a booger or rub your eyes, not to mention sticking your fingers in your mouth to dislodge a peanut.

Pets are also a lovely way to contract a world of hurt. Dogs and cats will roll in feces, sniff up urine tracts and then bring home dead animals in their mouth, only to ask you to pet them and fill your fingernails with microscopic organisms and then lick your face for good measure. If you are not washing your hands after holding your hamster or hound dog, then you are just asking for nasty sickness.

I'm not going to go into all of the sorted types of diarrhea that can plague you from lack of hygiene, or the zillion types of organisms that can nest *under* your skin. But if this book does nothing more than get you to keep your body clean and tidy, then it has done a lot.

I celebrate our society's explosion of personal-care services that foster health and wellness. These things will impact your general sense of good health and personal confidence. It should go without saying that if you indulge in the services of any personal care facility, be sure to note the hygiene of the employees, who should be sterilizing combs, wearing gloves and cleaning instruments. Many people have received infections from nail salons that fail to sterilize their equipment before shoving it under your cuticles and nails.

Speaking of which, manicures and pedicures remain among the most popular personal-care services. Many of my friends view their painted nails as a mere byproduct of the amazing foot and hand massages that they receive there. My male friends also swear by these finger and toe treatments. I see almost as many men in the chairs as I see women.

Full and partial body massages have also migrated from the world of high-end resorts to affordable, monthly or weekly budget items. Franchise massage services are popping up in every strip mall and can be accessed for as little as $25 per massage. In addition to providing a feeling of overall wellbeing, it will help you relax when life starts to send you damaging stress.

Joint adjustments are a similar indulgence that falls under personal care. If you have serious back issues, I recommend seeing your doctor and getting referred to a specialist, but for simple tightness in the back or neck, many are adding their local joint-adjuster to their regular regimen.

I once read about one of the leading NBA basketball players, who would go to the chiropractor *four times* on game days. While that is extreme for most of us, it allowed him to succeed in his career. Another friend of mine vacationed at a resort that included massage twice a day.

I know many men who invest in hot shaves before important meetings or big events. Today, men's grooming shops have propagated, providing a host of rejuvenating skin treatments, pore-tightening tonics and dirt-removing exfoliation services. As women have known for years, facial treatments promote health and wellbeing.

If money is tight, there are a million home-application facials and mud treatments that come in single-use packets that can be bought for a few dollars at neighborhood pharmacies or discount department stores. Home therapies even include aromatherapy with high tech essential oil diffusers that can be found at the mall, online or even some grocery stores. Feeling well can lead to *being* well.

When I got married, my cousin Robert Patton, who has spent his entire career in the healthcare industry, gave us a folding massage table along with a gift certificate for massage classes. I don't have to tell you that a folding massage table is the gift that keeps on giving.

It is just like the professional ones, and now we have a whole set of amazing oils and potions that provide life-giving treatments. I even bought some of those fake flickering candles and a pack of $15 massage stones that can be heated. Talk about *relationship therapy* too. Within five minutes, my wife and I can set up the table, flip on the candles, launch a Zen music app and settle into our own home spa.

I confess that just a few years ago, I discovered the world of body waxing. But, before you applaud my bravery or decry my vanity, I have to say that the verdict is out on the health benefits of waxing. Today there are waxing salons on every corner offering different kinds of products and procedures. It's the rage for many good reasons, but simply assuming that hair is gross should not be one of them. Some people associate hair with oil and smell and one more thing to wash. The truth is that while you must keep all hair clean, hair grows in places for a reason. It often acts as a trap or filter for allergens, pollutants and other airborne transmitters of ill health. Nose hairs keep out all kinds of bacteria, as do eyebrows and eyelashes.

Whitney Bowe, MD, is a dermatologist in Briarcliff Manor, New York, and clinical assistant professor of dermatology at Mount Sinai Medical School in New York City. He says that our hair "acts as a shield against bacteria, allergens, and other unwanted pathogens." He also says that stripping away that natural barrier puts you at higher risk of irritation or infection, especially when it comes to STDs.

A study conducted by San Francisco General Hospital tracked 7,500 people who were sexually active and found that those who shaved their genital regions were 400 percent more likely to get STDs. It is important to note that this may be attributed to a number of factors, ranging from tiny skin cuts that opened up pathways for transmitting disease, to possibly the fact that those who waxed were simply having more sex. Just remember that if you have hair anywhere, keep it clean.

If, on the other hand, waxing makes you feel healthier and sexier, then I vote for proceeding with reasonable caution, and a commitment to monitor your hairless dermis. In some cases, you can reduce the *amount* of hair without having to rip it out. It's called shaving.

Lastly, I must mention the meteoric rise of yoga, Pilates and barre. These are all amazing self-care ways to stretch, strengthen and reduce stress. I have done yoga and even hot yoga and barely survived. They are definitely not for the timid, but can greatly benefit the heart, mind and body. They can be a great alternative to the gym if you use them to increase your heart rate and build muscle. Moreover, they are great ways to get connected to a community of healthy people. I know a lot of people who will go to their yoga class because it is their friend group. It is their connection time with likeminded people who value health and wellness.

Earlier, I advocated for joining a gym and, fortunately, a lot of gyms offer yoga or similar stretching and strengthening classes, as well as cardio, dance and weight classes so you can have the best of both worlds by joining one place.

Either way, making such disciplines part of your *daily* physical activity routine is the way to make it a brainless activity so that you can reap the benefits that only come from routine behavior. And remember, when you're in the gym or yoga studio, use hand sanitizer. It's brainless.

CHAPTER TWENTY

WEALTH HEALTH

FOR SOME, THIS IS the chapter that they've been waiting for and the reason they bought the book. They are looking for the secrets to avoid spiraling into financial ruin. Good news; not only can you dodge the financial flames, you can *make money* while improving your health.

Financial stress can be a monster health killer. Think Godzilla. That's because financial stress causes the body to release multiple stress hormones such as cortisol and adrenalin. Your blood, your organs and even your skin are being mercilessly attacked, and they can't last long before suffering irreparable damage.

According to the Hormone Health Network (See: hormone.org) the following can happen:

- Stomach pains, due to a slow-down in the rate that the stomach empties after eating; also, diarrhea due to more activity in the colon.

- Increase in excessive appetite, which will lead to weight gain and of course puts you at risk for diabetes and cardiovascular disease.

- Weakened immune system so that you are more likely to have colds, inflammation and infections.

- Anxiety, depression, loss of sleep, and lack of interest in being active. Memory and decision-making can also be affected.

- Increase in blood pressure, heart rate, and the level of fats in your blood (cholesterol and triglycerides). Also, increases in blood sugar levels.

All these result in heightened risk for heart disease, hardening of the arteries, stroke, obesity, and diabetes.

These physical manifestations don't even begin to address the way that stress affects our relationships. We become jerks at home and work. We are obnoxious to those we love, start to retreat from others and withdraw in general from all social environments. Our work suffers, and people start to respond to us with irritation, which exacerbates stress and frustration.

According to the Institute for Divorce Financial Analysts, *money issues* rank third behind infidelity and incompatibility as reasons for divorce. Among other things, financial worry leads to overall worry, which in turn contributes to poor sleep. Sleeplessness increases one's susceptibility to illness and irritability, which simply fuels the circle of stress. Everyone suffers. Lastly, one's ability to make logical and prudent decisions diminishes, which leads to even more financial screwups. It is not uncommon for people who are financially stressed to *spend more* money that they don't have. They run up credit cards with meals out, drinking, entertainment and even shopping sprees, in an irrational effort to calm their emotional distress.

Think of poor finances as the plague of death, the ultimate war against your health. If you cannot get a grip on your finances, your health will plummet out of control.

Throughout this book, I've tried to make it clear that health does not have to cost any more than ill health. In nearly every case, healthy choices will not only *cost less*, you can *make money* on the money you save. Therefore, if you find yourself in a downward financial spiral, double down on your health. I personally did so when I had zero resources.

There was a time in my life when I lost my wife, my home, my job and every single penny of savings and retirement, all at the same time, which quickly led to over $100,000 in debt and a crushing emotional state. While looking for work and a place to live, I hit the gym daily, and church every Sunday.

The only two financial expenses that were not up for negotiation were my Starbucks black coffee habit and my gym membership. To say that stress attacked me every single day for three years is a major understatement. But my determination to exercise had two equally powerful effects. It cleared my body of toxic stress while increasing my self-confidence.

I was sweating out toxins from my body while releasing hormones, like dopamine, which improved my mood and outlook. While I was continually reaching new personal bests in the gym, by running further or lifting more weight, I was showing myself that I could overcome obstacles. I was proving to myself that I could improve myself. These physical accomplishments helped me believe that I could overcome my emotional and financial challenges.

On top of that, I looked better, felt better, and those around me noticed. That in turn led me to perform better in interviews and more easily establish new friendships and romantic interests. It even gave me greater confidence and clarity to deal with creditors and build money saving strategies that helped me dig out one dollar at a time.

The bottom line is that my daily commitment to my health was a huge catalyst to my overall stabilization, financially and otherwise.

PRACTICAL ADVICE

The link that humans have toward money is almost as powerful as it is toward food and sex. We love making and spending money. Unfortunately, we are not as in love with saving money. It's not as much fun for most. So how can financial health be brainless?

First, we must adopt two competing principles. One is *scarcity* and the other is *abundance*. If you do much reading in the areas of finances or personal self-help, you will discover that one or the other of these principles are typically embraced. Not here. *I believe in embracing them both.*

Scarcity is of course the idea that you only have so much money and you might run out. That's perfectly normal and can be completely healthy if taken in the right context. It is normal because at any given point in time it is 100 percent true. Your bank account has a fixed amount of money, making it a fixed asset. Secondly, no one can control the future, which means that you could lose your money in a flash due to identity theft, job loss, market crash, or global war.

That reality should cause you to recognize the need for saving at least one or two pieces of your financial pie for later. Sock it away somewhere super safe like an insured savings account or similar institutional account.

The concept of *abundance* speaks to the idea that you can always make more financial pies and that having more pieces of pie will protect you when times get tough. Most people can earn more money *if they believe* that there are always more ways to earn money.

Perhaps it is by adding a second job. Maybe it is simply the ability to earn more money at your current job. Regardless, you must believe that there is an *abundance of money* hiding inside an *abundance of opportunities.*

By embracing both scarcity and abundance, you can greatly improve your financial health and in turn improve your physical health. You will have additional money to spend on your health, from fitness to healthy food to vacations, and you will sleep better, behave better and think better because you know that you have some money tucked away for a rainy day or even an outright monsoon.

Start by making a habit of withdrawing money from your checking account on a regular basis and stashing it away. Yep. Even if you are living paycheck to paycheck and stretching every dollar, still take out *some money* on a disciplined, regular basis.

If you have an employer who will allow you to split your direct deposit paycheck, this is the simplest brainless option. You will have to set up a separate savings account at your bank or a different bank and then tell your employer to send a specific percentage or dollar amount from each paycheck into your savings account and direct the rest to your normal checking account. You will never need to think about saving again. It will just grow and grow and grow. You will never see the money in your checking account and so you will be forced to budget on what remains.

Personally, I like the discipline of going to the ATM. I love touching the cold hard cash. It's as basic as that. I pick a specific time like every Friday or every Saturday morning. I go to the ATM and withdraw $100 and stick it in a coffee can. If you don't have much money to deduct, then don't deduct much money. Take out as much as you can afford to take out *on a regular basis.* Don't take out $500 one time and then $10 the next. That takes too much thinking to calculate how much you can afford or what bills are about to come due. The brainless key is a consistent amount on a consistent, predicable, automatic schedule.

My favorite place to stash cash is in an empty wine bottle. That's because it will likely require me to break the bottle in order to get it out and spend it. The idea of course is not to spend it under any circumstances, and believe me the wine bottle typically does the trick.

I love this tactic because most of us like to *see and feel* actual money. It's soothing going to bed at night knowing that you have a coffee can or wine bottle stuffed with $2,000. It feels better than seeing an electronic bank statement. Moreover, no one is going to hack your wine bottle. However, be sure to hide it in your home in case your home gets robbed. You don't want it conspicuously on the counter with dollar bills coming out of the bottle neck.

To really fatten that nest egg, make a habit of applying for jobs or side gigs. An old business principle says that you can make *more* money either by finding new customers or getting more out of the ones you already have. It's that simple.

So, start by asking for a raise. You don't need to fret over it or fear that your boss will get mad at you for asking. If anything, they will be the ones who get scared thinking that you are looking for more money and might quit. So, don't sweat it.

Just walk in and say, "Hey, I was wondering if I could get a raise in my pay?" Then they will take it from there. If they don't say yes, then hopefully they will give you a path for you to follow to earn a raise in the future.

In the event the boss does not embrace your request, you need to make a habit of applying for jobs on LinkedIn or other job websites *every Wednesday morning before 8 a.m.* According to zipjob.com, Tuesday through Thursday is statistically the optimum time to send in a resume in order to avoid getting caught in the Monday morning crush or the Friday afternoon signoff. Hubspot.com tracked twenty million emails over ten months and confirmed this.

It was also noted that sending a resume late at night or early in the morning is best, but I advocate the early morning for two reasons. First, it shows that you are an early riser and that you work hard in the morning. Second, there are a lot of spam emails sent late at night, and you want your resume to arrive after the hiring manager deletes all the junk in the morning.

You can even write the email at night and hit send when you wake up in the morning. It's as easy as that. The point is that you have to go *job fishing* every week, rain or shine. Remember that *you never have to take a job. But you cannot take a job if it is never offered to you.* Just do it for the experience of writing cover letters and perfecting your communication. And, if you do it while you are still employed, you will be far less stressed and appear far less desperate if and when you get the interview. You will be able to relax and be yourself.

In the case that you love your job but there is no money for a raise, then it is time to start hunting for *extra* side work. Imagine what an extra $100, $200 or $1,000 a month would do for you. Seriously, stop and imagine it. That can be achieved very easily. It might mean an extra family night out to the movies or an extra vacation to the beach. It doesn't have to rule your life, but it might be fun to have some extra spending dough.

I support the idea that if you are going to spend more of your time working beyond your regular hours, do something that you are either good at or something that you really like. The first step is to find out what you are good at, from gardening to building websites to doing social media to painting. Then simply ask Google how to start a gardening side business or how to start a painting company or how make money walking dogs. You get the point. I know a guy who makes $200,000 a year walking dogs.

Once you start to squirrel away savings (the principle of scarcity) and expand your earning potential (the principle of abundancy) your financial health will improve little by little and your overall health will skyrocket overnight. That's because you will feel more secure and more hopeful, which will be felt in your sleep and in your relationships. Trust me. Do it today. Don't delay, because if you wait until you are desperate, it might be too late. Your health will already be under siege and it will be far harder to maintain either habit.

INVEST IN HEALTH SAVINGS

This is not an investing book. There are eight million books on that subject. Get one of those books and follow their simple strategies. My job is to convince you that finances and health go hand in hand.

Just to nail the point home in practical terms, if someone who smokes a pack a day decides to invest his/her $10-a-day death habit into the stock market and averaged 6 percent annual interest compounded daily, after thirty years the former smoker would be sitting on $305,876 in cash, and breathing a heck of a lot better.

You can do the same financial magic with all kinds of things. Go check out David Bach's brilliant *latte factor* calculator at https://davidbach.com/latte-factor/. Instead of cigarettes, put in something else that you can cut back on. Maybe it's not every day but just on weekends. Maybe it is one less drink at the bar on Friday and Saturday night every week. That could easily be a $20 savings every week. If you invested just the money that you would have spent on those two extra drinks per week, you'd have $87,153 in thirty years.

If you must drink alcohol, consider inviting your friends over to your house and pouring them drinks from *your own* bar. Buying your own booze by the bottle will make you a hit with your friends and you will end up spending *far less* money than at the bar.

Maybe you can start investing the money that you save from that weekly bag of potato chips at the grocery store. Instead of buying that item, you are going to take that whopping $3.89 and dump it into an investment account every week and watch it grow. In thirty years, when the kids are grown, you can fly to the Maldives or Fiji or Egypt in first class and stay at a five-star resort on the $17,000 that those former potato chips earned you. And of course, your body will be way healthier as a result of cutting back on those chips over the years. It's brainless to save, invest and feel better as a result.

EATING IN

A friend of mine once told me, "When you eat out, you hand over your health *and your wallet*." I love that phrase because it is 100 percent true. You have no idea what oil or ingredients they used to cook your food or what quality of food they purchased for your meal. On top of handing over control of what exactly you are eating and how it is cooked, you are paying them top dollar for potential ill health. Today, the cost of eating out is at least twice if not three times what it would be if you dined at home. Especially if you include tip, taxes and parking.

Don't get me wrong, I enjoy eating out. I consider it entertainment. I'd rather go out to eat than go to the movies. But when I needed to improve my financial health, it was a luxury that I could not afford.

Start cooking in your own kitchen for your physical health, and your wallet will get healthier too. Recently, our family decided to make up a restaurant name for our own kitchen. We tell the kids, "We are going to eat at Club 870 for dinner tonight." It's goofy, but it makes it fun and it ups our game with regard to what we cook and how we serve it. We light candles, turn on the music, etc.

If you really want to have some fun with eating in, go to the grocery store and buy your favorite gourmet dinner ingredients for *one meal.* Buy the steak you love or buy the gourmet pizza. Buy a bottle of wine or pick up some shrimp cocktail appetizer. And don't forget dessert. Grab a single pint, or half-pint, of gourmet ice cream or one of those single slices of pie. Spare no expense on that single meal. Tally it up at the register and I guarantee it will be at least half what you would have paid at a restaurant for the exact same items. It's mind numbing. It's fun. You can eat a $100 meal for $35 or less, easily.

I've even done that when I feel like indulging at a sports bar with some wings and beer. Instead, I'll hit the grocery store and stock up on buffalo wings that just need heating and the exact same beer I would order at the bar. All of it costs *less than half* the price of the bar, and I get a six-pack of beer for the cost of a single beer at the bar. It's insane.

If you want to really seal the deal, try transferring the money that you saved by going to the grocery store instead of the restaurant to your savings account right on your phone's banking app after you finish at the grocery register. Seriously, go into your bank account and transfer your best estimate of the difference that you think you would have paid at a restaurant. Believe me, you will enjoy your meal even more.

AVOID ILLNESS

Simple medications for the flu, a cold, allergies or other illnesses can cost a staggering amount. Eating healthy at home can save gobs of money by keeping you healthy.

Recently a plumber came to visit my friend's house. He saw her cooking a healthy meal of vegetables and he told her that he changed his diet 180 degrees three years ago and now he eats vegetables every day. She asked why; and he told her that he was diagnosed with diabetes. He said that it wasn't the disease diagnosis that motivated him to change his ways, it was that he realized that the insulin would run him a minimum of $600/month, *after* insurance. He knew he didn't have that money to spare. He said it was a heck of a lot cheaper to fix his menu. Predictably, he lost fifty pounds and completely reversed his diabetes so that he needs zero medicine now. The kicker was that he said he never knew how delicious and fun healthy eating could be.

I have countless stories like that. One of my friends used to take antacids every single night. Then one day he changed his diet and his weight went down. His sleep went up and his antacids went completely away. I have often wished that I could give people a glimpse of how a healthy body feels. I really think if people knew what they were forfeiting by eating metaphorical Pop-Tarts and Twinkies, they'd change in a minute.

Few people stop and take the time to calculate the cost for insulin, blood pressure medicine or a cholesterol drug. Most people have no idea what medicines cost until they are prescribed them. Even fewer people can imagine the cost of multiple medications. Can you believe the financial stress you would be under if you suddenly had to add a slew of meds to your monthly budget? It's NUTS. I have a friend who pays a psychiatrist a ton of money to help her kid with hyperactivity while at the same time she still feeds him pounds of sugar from juices, sodas, cookies and muffins. There are health expenses that are completely avoidable. When I brush my teeth, I do it with dollar signs running through my head. I don't want to pay for cavities and crowns if I can avoid it.

I want everyone to wake up in the morning, no matter how much money they have, and say, "I absolutely cannot afford to get sick. That's not where I'm going to spend my money." Prevent, prevent, prevent so you can play, play, play and save, save, save. Today it might be cough syrup and allergy pills. Tomorrow it might be prescription drugs and the next day it could be an oxygen tank or dialysis. This is not a joke. It's no exaggeration. One in five Americans are sent to collections for medical bills. Many of those could have been completely avoided. Completely. Stay healthy and save gobs of money. What could be more brainless?

My heart breaks in a thousand pieces for those filing for bankruptcy because of a disease or disability that could *not* be avoided. Imagine, one day you are saving for retirement and the next day a tractor trailer rear-ends you or some rare bacteria, virus or cancer attacks you from out of nowhere. Suddenly, you are handing over every penny you have to some hospital or insurance company. I cannot imagine the millions of families that are eating peanut butter and jelly today because they sent every dollar to the hospital. I can only say that we all are one phone call away from hearing that we have a terminal illness and that treatment will cost hundreds of thousands of dollars. Whenever we have the chance, we need to impress upon our elected officials that healthcare reform is way overdue.

Lastly, I must mention a controversial, nasty little fact about health and wealth. Various studies correlate how much you earn to how much you weigh. In 2010, a landmark study was conducted by Dan Cable of the London School of Economics and Timothy Judge of the University of Florida. Together, they collected weight and income on over 20,000 people that revealed up to a $15,000 difference in pay between healthy weight individuals and those who were overweight. (Judge & Cable. *Journal of Applied Psychology*. 2010.)

This study, along with many others indicate a deep-seated cultural discrimination based on body weight. "There are several decades of research evidence demonstrating weight bias in the context of employment, and what we see is evidence of bias at essentially every stage of the hiring and employment cycle," reported Dr. Rebecca Puhl, deputy director of the University of Connecticut's Rudd Center for Food Policy & Obesity.

It gets worse. According to these studies, overweight people are seen as less conscientious, less productive, lazy, lacking in self-discipline, and even dishonest.

Discrimination of any kind is disgusting. There are hundreds of reasons that someone might be overweight that go far beyond their ability to control. To blame or punish them for it is the highest form of ignorance and cruelty.

Now add the topic of health to the issue and you have an even bigger problem. That's because there is far less data on workplace discrimination based on *health issues* than weight issues, and I believe it's far more rampant.

Why do I know it? Because it's logical. Productivity is money. Health issues take you out of the office. They take you out of the game. You can't work when you are sick. Moreover, you often take time off to go to the doctor and even go back to the doctor for follow-up visits. Just one bout with the flu is a major cost to your employer. Imagine employees who are constantly getting sick, let alone those with chronic illnesses.

Even if you manage to hide your illnesses during the interview, they can still be a real threat to your chances for advancement, your overall earning potential and even keeping your job. No one is going to tell you that because it is illegal. That's why I'm here.

I haven't even mentioned the financial hard costs that companies incur related to employee sickness and the medical claims that they generate ranging from medical procedures to prescriptions. I'm always blown away by employees who don't understand the cost connection between employee health and cost to their company. Way too many employees assume insurance companies magically pick up the cost of their lack of health. They never sit down and think about the fact that their employer is either paying for their medical bills directly or doing so via higher and higher insurance premiums.

Healthcare is the number one cost for most employers. According to Integrated Benefits Institute president Thomas Parry, "The cost of poor health to employers is greater than the combined revenues of Apple, Amazon, Microsoft, Netflix, eBay and Adobe."

That's why smart employers are falling all over themselves to hand out Fitbits and jump ropes. Believe me, they are not rolling out wellness programs and offering gym memberships because they suddenly thought it was a nice thing to do. They are doing so in hopes of saving millions of dollars in medical claims. If one person gets diabetes, the company is going to take a hit. According to the American Diabetes Association, "People with diagnosed diabetes incur average medical expenditures of $16,752 per year. People with diagnosed diabetes, on average, have medical expenditures approximately 2.3 times higher than what expenditures would be in the absence of diabetes."

Pause for a minute and consider that massive number. Sure, I'm talking about the cost to employers, but with every chunk of change your employer is paying, you are paying a ton as well. The fastest way to secure your current paycheck while shrinking your own bills is to get as healthy as possible, and stay that way.

Despite federal laws protecting patient privacy, most organizations know who's healthy and who's not. They know who is costing the company tons of money in terms of medical claims and who's not. How do I know? Think about it. They listen at the water cooler. They hear how you spent your weekend. They know who signs up for the company 5K run and who doesn't. They see what you munch on at your desk and what you eat at the company picnic or office birthday parties. Plus, health information tends to fall out of our conversations. People are quick to share plenty of health information about their bad back, their bum knee or their headaches with coworkers.

Conversely, healthy people might reveal that they have started taking probiotics or read a news article about sunscreen. They might mention that they joined a gym or that the gym is crowded after work. Perhaps the biggest health topic that populates the collective conversation is that of diets. People love to talk about their new diet or how they have started eating salads or tofu or less red meat. We talk about what is important to us and we don't talk about what is not. Pretty basic. Pretty revealing.

Furthermore, as a health communicator, I know that when it comes to health messaging, one size does not fit all. People are motivated by a million different things, and if you are motivated by a bigger paycheck or a chance to score the corner office, I'm fine with that. I honestly don't care what causes you to get your ass healthy. Just do it.

CHAPTER TWENTY-ONE

STRETCHING BODY, MIND, SPIRIT

I ADMIT THAT THE topic of "stretching" is not completely brainless. A lot of people have no idea how to stretch other than the natural kind that they do when they yawn in the morning. Maybe they learned to touch their toes in elementary school, but that's about it. Of course, YouTube has no lack of videos to help you stretch like Gumby, and that part is completely brainless. So, start surfing the net.

Similarly, when it comes to stretching the mind and spirit, there are far too many ways to *stretch* than I could ever list in this book. Entire categories of books have been dedicated to mindfulness, meditation and prayer, not to mention stillness, yoga and self-talk.

Regardless, I couldn't leave out the topic of stretching because of the critical health benefits associated with stretching every fiber in your body, mind and soul.

STAYING STRETCHY

When it comes to the body, Healthline.com cites a National Institutes of Health report that shows that stretching increases circulation, which improves blood flow to the muscles that in turn improve recovery time and muscle soreness due to exercise. Additionally, they say that stretching can prevent back pain by reducing stiffness. We've all reached in the backseat of our car and felt a tweak in our back. It happens opening a jar of pickles, reaching in the closet or picking up a suitcase.

To that end, as good as YouTube videos are, if you can afford to get guidance from a physical therapist, personal trainer or other health professional, then definitely do it. Regardless, go slow and try not to pull anything in the process. Try stretching *after* a hot shower. Get the water nice and hot, and then after you get out, do a little stretching. Typically, the hot water will have loosened up your muscles just enough to provide a little extra flexibility.

Then, once you have a little routine of stretches developed, build them into your daily discipline and enjoy the endless benefits, which according to some medical professionals include a reduction in headaches, improvement in posture and overall calmness. I don't know about all of that, but the bottom line is that you won't suffer from staying stretchy.

TAKE YOUR BRAIN TO THE GYM

When it comes to stretching your mind, you absolutely need to get busy. The mind needs to work out almost as much as your body. When we are young, our mind learns constantly. People say that young minds are like a sponges but the fact is that we desperately need information, so our mind is on a mission to absorb, process and categorize trillions of tiny pieces of information like how to walk, talk and eat, how to go to school, socialize, and watch TV. Each interaction or form of communication teaches us exponentially more until one day, we get fat and happy with what we know and slow our learning.

We drive the same way to work. Listen to the same music. We watch the same TV shows. Some people even watch the same shows and movies *again and again*. We hang out with the same people and speak the same language, using the same set of words that we already know. How many people do you know who actively try to increase their vocabulary? Many people do the same tasks at their job and they pack the same lunches, go to the same restaurants, vacation in the same places. In short, we stop stimulating our brains. We stop learning for the most part. You will even hear people say that they *can't handle* any more information. You hear the term *information overload*, and a lot of people believe we can overfill our brains. I'm not a neurologist, but there's no way I'm buying into that hooey.

Then, change comes. Big or small. We lose our job or our kids leave the house or we get sick. Suddenly, we must start learning again, and it can be as challenging as exercising our bodies after years of sitting around. After a while, we even begin to *forget* stuff. We forget how to play the piano, or we forget how to speak the foreign language that we learned in school. We forget names and can't remember dates. Sure, the mind ages just like the body, *and just like the body* it will age quicker and with greater severity if it is not exercised.

Today there are so many ways to exercise your brain. You are never too old to learn a musical instrument or a foreign language. You can read books that will stretch your mind and send it to places it never dreamed of going. Books can be like traveling without ever leaving your home. They will transport you, and your brain will be ignited to think thoughts completely beyond the content of the book itself. Books are like fire starters. Today, you can listen to audio books or even write your own book. It doesn't have to be a best seller but could be just for your kids or grandkids. You can learn to bake new foods, candy or mix exotic cocktails. You can start a company or help someone start one. You can mentor someone or become someone's mentee. You can make new friends, join new clubs, volunteer, garden, or learn to build your own mobile app. I venture to guess that there is nothing that you endeavor to learn that you can't learn online for zero money. The internet is the ultimate teaching machine.

I am a lover of the library. For me, it is like a candy store. I used to take my kids to the library and tell them to pick out any book they wanted about something to learn. Sometimes it was a makeup book or a cookbook or a book on war. Sometimes they chose books about dating or dogs or the jungle. The library is different than the internet because online you have to type exactly what you want in order to see. Add to that, it will only return results that are related to your search, but in a library, you get to visually scan a book about motorcycles right next to one on monsters or the Maldives. In the author section, you get even more diversity. It is so much fun because you can take the book home, flip through it and use one recipe or one hairstyle and then return it, all for free. Try it with your kids and yourself. Stretch your brain.

I listen to Spanish tutorials while I'm on the treadmill. I watch YouTube videos about how to build websites and I read instructional blogs about how to use my fancy new camera. I stretch and stretch and stretch my brain. I Google recipes when I cook and enter the craft beers I drink into an app. Finally, I try to learn how to take my social media to the next level so that I can reach more and more people about brainless health. That's just for starters.

My mom used to say that "curiosity killed the cat." I don't believe that curiosity kills anything. *I think curiosity is the great protector.* It is the great preserver of the gray matter between our ears. Stay curious. Stay interested. The verdict is currently out as to whether we can stave off Alzheimer's and other cognitive disorders by exercising our brain, but as for me, I'm certainly going to die trying.

Visit, speak, hear, taste, read, calculate, invent, dream, view and experience as many new things as often as possible. It will feel uncomfortable, so expect that and do it anyway. Keep learning, thinking, questioning and doing. At very least it will make you a way more interesting person to be around.

STRETCH YOUR SPIRIT

I took a trip to Alaska where I flew over glaciers, hiked to waterfalls and lakes, took a train and then a boat to see the fjords, saw crazy amounts of wildlife and utterly spectacular sunsets. When I watch rushing river water that never stops, yet allows food to grow, and plant life to thrive under its current, I am amazed. Or if I ponder our atmosphere that is precisely calibrated to support teeming microscopic life inside lichens, urchins and even rocks that exist miles beneath the earth's surface, it gives me pause. Various gases and air particles present beautiful, changing colors, layers and even scents. For goodness sakes, just the twenty-two feet of rising tide that flows into Anchorage's Turnagain Arm and recedes every day based on the moon is enough to leave me speechless. But that's not all. Just consider the glacial silt that looks like pure mud, but in fact is completely healthy to drink. The silt is so fine and full of minerals that if you set a jar of it on your windowsill, the silt will never settle. That's crazy amazing.

Have you ever thought about the relationship between salmon and zooplankton? According to NASA's website *earthdata* (https://earthdata.nasa.gov/learn/sensing-our-planet/boom-or-bust-the-bond-between-fish-and-phytoplankton), "The marine food chain starts with microscopic plants called phytoplankton, which typically float close to the surface where there is sunlight for photosynthesis. Phytoplankton are eaten by slightly larger, more mobile, herbivores called zooplankton, which range in size from single-celled organisms to jellyfish. In turn, zooplankton provide food for krill and salmon."

Think about that the next time you order salmon at a restaurant, or the fact that 80 million salmon spawn every single year, just in Alaska.

Imagine the research about the precise purpose of a lion's mane or the quills of a porcupine or the translucent bodies of cave crawfish. Nature screams at me every day. It stands in defiance of my own abilities and knowledge. It shades me, gives me oxygen (uses my exhalation to grow fifty-foot trees), provides me with plants and animals that have the perfect nutrition for my body, circadian sleep patterns from the moon, water to hydrate my organs and seasonal colors to delight the retinas of my eyes. I appreciate those who say that they do not believe in anything beyond themselves but are still burdened by what they cannot explain. If there is nothing more than myself, then I am the end-all-be-all of everything. I must come up with explanations for everything that happens or doesn't happen. That puts a ton of stress on the body and the brain, because a lot in life simply doesn't make sense outside of a larger faith paradigm.

In my research, I found study after study that discussed spiritually devout people having fewer symptoms of depression and anxiety, as well as a better ability to cope with stress. Some studies suggest that spiritual/religious practices may even change the brain in a way that increases mental health.

I personally believe in a loving God that created me and whose son cares to have a relationship with me. That foundational truth in my life influences everything I do, say and think. It drives my motivation, my morality, my work ethic, the way I approach relationships, the way I treat people, the way I spend, save and share my money, the commitments I make or don't make and the extremely high value that I place on my health. Believe me, it's not about being pure or holy or perfect or better than anyone else, but it does make me better at life compared to when I didn't have faith. I think it also makes me better at friendship and fatherhood and *husbandhood*. It provides me with peace and purpose and hope, which in turn helps me sleep at night and wake up in the morning with expectation instead of dread.

Today, spiritualism, spiritism, spirituality, religiosity or just plain religion are multi-dimensional terms that carry a lot of historical and cultural baggage. Words and labels and titles can get in the way of the potential health benefits of believing in someone or something greater than yourself. It is undeniable that every human being must wonder, at least once in their life, where they came from and where they are going. That tiny question causes many people to search in every corner of the universe, internet, temple, church or bookstore to find a satisfying answer. I believe that the quest to discover your place and purpose can be deeply healthful. It is a journey, and I believe that any journey can be full of excitement, adventure, purpose and expectation. Even after faith is discovered, it typically ignites an ongoing journey that never ends. Faith, or even a search for faith, is far from brainless.

The part that *is* brainless is that faith doesn't hurt. If you believe in something bigger than yourself, then everyone wins. Everything begins to have a purpose. You start to invest in your community and strangers that you don't even know. You support kids and the homeless and the sick, because it aligns with your beliefs. Suddenly your family matters more. You begin to think about legacy. I personally don't know if everything happens for a reason, but I firmly believe that God has a plan for everyone. For me, it is more intellectually satisfying to turn to my faith when bizarre things happen instead of simply chalking it up to coincidence or chance. Like I always say, it would take more faith for me to believe in hundreds of coincidences than to believe in my God.

When it comes to brainlessness, listening to sermons or homilies or messages, or reading inspired literature, or listening to theological teachers, typically provides great lessons and tactics for dealing with *life in general.* Solid spiritual teaching usually provides insights and instruction to life's practical challenges, such as handling conflict at work, financial fears and of course dealing with serious health issues. I tell people that they should come to church with me and learn clever ways to parent, handle holiday stress, be financially responsible or treat the body with respect. It's always a no-brainer to avail yourself of smart people, regardless of what you believe.

Even the US Department of Defense recognizes the value of *spiritual fitness* when it comes to readiness. According to the DOD's website, "Total Force Fitness is a holistic concept for building and maintaining health, readiness, and optimal performance of the US

Armed Forces using the connection between mind, body, spirit, environment and relationships." They have discovered that a wheel doesn't work well if one of the spokes is missing.

Of course, Alcoholics Anonymous is famous for making faith in a higher power the foundation of their twelve-step process. There are a gazillion additional examples where faith is foundational. I think it is simply nuts not to tap into its potential.

I haven't even mentioned the benefits of meditation, prayer or stillness that often accompany every flavor of faith. If only to carve out some quiet time in an age of communication assault, you can't help but benefit. As I mentioned earlier, there are scores of audio, video and printed materials to assist with this, and I soundly support anything that gives your spirit a respite. Even breathing techniques, mindfulness or sitting still will change your pulse. Frankly, if you only develop a daily discipline of *silence* to gather your thoughts before work or reviewing your to-do list, you will still benefit immensely.

So, whether you already have faith or are considering the search, stretch your spirt.

CHAPTER TWENTY-TWO

WATER, FREEBIES AND LABELS

I DON'T HAVE TIME or enough pages left to dig into these three additional topics, but it's critical that you adhere to them. Think of them like bonus tips. They are as brainless as everything else in this book, so please lock them into your brain and throw away the key.

DRINK UP

At least in the United States, every time you sit down at a restaurant, the waiter brings you a glass of water. Drink it. Just about every office, health club, mattress store or Jiffy Lube® has a water cooler. Take a cup. Sixty percent of your body is made up of water. The United States Geological Survey (usgs.gov) reports that according to H. H. Mitchell in the *Journal of Biological Chemistry*, the brain and heart are composed of 73 percent water, and the lungs about 83 percent. The skin contains 64 percent water, muscles and kidneys are 79 percent, and even the bones are watery at 31 percent. When you don't properly hydrate, your skin, kidneys, lungs, heart and brain suffer.

Think about your house plants. You go on vacation and they shrivel up. You water them and they almost miraculously spring back to life. It's amazing to see it. But those house plants are a tiny indicator of exactly what happens to your body when you water it. Think of drinking water as watering your *bodyplant*. It's so simple, so brainless and so super full of health. You will think better, work better, play better and sleep better. And it is so simple. I went to IKEA and got one of these super cool glass liter water bottles with a cork top for a dollar. I fill it up, stick it in the fridge, and whenever I open the fridge (800 times a day) I see it and take a swig as if I were a pirate and it was a bottle of rum! It's always there. Always cold. Always satisfying. Completely brainless.

GET YOUR FREE DOCTOR VISIT

Mom and Dad taught me that there is never a free lunch, but fortunately, there is a free physician checkup every year. Put it on the calendar. Treat it like your birthday or anniversary. Don't miss it. It is the best gift that you can give yourself or your family. Treat it like Tax Day or Christmas or Halloween. Simply put it on the calendar like a fixed, full-moon, annual event.

In case you happened to miss the biggest healthcare debate in American history, you can now receive an *annual checkup free of cost*, as part of the Affordable Care Act. This law guarantees a slew of other preventive services for men, women and children, so take a gander at the government's website to find other freebies.

Women: https://www.healthcare.gov/preventive-care-women/

Children: https://www.healthcare.gov/preventive-care-children/

Adults: https://www.healthcare.gov/preventive-care-adults/

It doesn't matter what insurance you have; *it's free*. You get the chance to meet with a doctor, ask questions and walk out of the office with the peace of mind that either nothing is wrong with you or that you are going to get some help to fix anything that *is* wrong. It's brainless if you really want to live the best possible life.

I knew a woman who worked in public health and was scared to death of going to the doctor. She had not gone to the doctor in nine years. I asked her when the last time she went and she replied, "When I had my baby." News flash, if you have a baby, then you absolutely, positively *owe it to your baby* to visit the doctor annually.

I told her straight up that she was playing Russian roulette with her life and the life of her child. To me, it is complete negligence for parents not to take care of themselves. Who's going to care for your kid if you are not alive and well? So, call up your doctor and schedule your annual exam pronto. If you don't have a primary care doctor, start calling to get one. With the help of Google and your insurance company's customer service number, you will find one. If you are still unsuccessful, drop by a pharmacy's help desk or outpatient center, such as CVS's Minute Clinic, and ask one of their docs how you can get your annual wellness checkup. They won't conduct it for you, but they will likely direct you.

DENTAL CLEANINGS

Unlike your annual physical checkup with your doctor, not everyone has dental insurance. Nevertheless, if you do have dental insurance, then annual (or twice a year) cleanings are typically free. As I mentioned earlier, nice teeth are part of a nice resume. Good teeth can help you win friends and climb the corporate ladder. It's just a fact that beautiful, clean teeth have immeasurable value.

But as we've discussed already, healthy teeth go far beyond looking good. Healthy teeth can prevent tons of nasty, life-sucking diseases.

Going to the dentist regularly is completely brainless because you get a goodie bag of free toothpaste and floss, while getting an actual medical exam. Today, dentists can even screen you for cancer while checking you for gum disease and cavities.

Lastly, did I mention that it was free? Free is still the absolute number one most effective marketing tactic. People love free. I love free. Take advantage of as many free things in life as possible, starting with a visit to your doctor and dentist.

READ FOOD LABELS

This really deserves an entire book devoted to showing the brainless healthy choices you can make if you simply turn over the items that you buy and look at the sugar and calorie count on the package. Sure, you can look at the list of vitamins and minerals or the protein and carbs, but at very, very least, check out the sugar and total calories (per serving). They will be related.

Why those two things you ask? Simply because excess sugar is linked to a zillion horrific diseases such as obesity, diabetes, heart disease and cancer, to say nothing of screwing up your brain and hormones. There are plenty of books written about the dangers of sugar, so if you don't trust me, please read up. Today, the average American consumes almost 152 pounds of sugar a year according to the New Hampshire Department of Health and Human Services. That is equal to three pounds of sugar consumed every single week.

The worst part is that sugar hides in insidious places. It masquerades under names such as dextrose, maltose, glucose, fructose, corn sweetener, honey, corn syrup, sucrose, sorghum syrup, sorbitol, lactose, molasses, fruit juice concentrate, etc. That laundry list means that it will not always show up in the ingredients under the name of sugar. The good news is that in the US, every packaged food has a label with a number next to the word *sugar*. Typically, you will find another number that lists *added sugar*. That's the real kicker. There just wasn't enough sugar in the granola to begin with, so they threw in some more to make it so yummy that you would eat ten times the amount.

Second to sugar, calories are my favorite metric of choice. Simply put, calories are units of energy. You eat them to gain energy and you burn them to expend energy. If you consume more than you burn, you suffer. The body will store the extra calories as fat cells that will surround your organs and wreak havoc with them. You get the point. Look out for sugar and calories.

So, the brainless part is simply flipping your products over before you buy them and checking out the sugar and calorie count listed on the back. Why is this brainless? Because very often, a different brand of the exact same product will be lower in sugar or lower in calories. I'm talking about flipping over a package of four tortillas or pita bread or ice cream or protein bars. Sometimes, just getting a different *flavor* of the exact same brand can have fewer sugar grams or calories. Why wouldn't you do this?

This has become a completely brainless habit of mine now. It is actually a game. I try to see how many calories and sugar grams I can cut, and still buy all the items on my grocery list. Of course, sometimes it forces me to not buy the product at all. If the sugar amount is 58 grams, like it is in a lot of "healthy" juices, I won't even consider it. When I find obscene amounts of sugar, I post them on my SugarFixChallenge Instagram page (@SugarFixChallenge). It blows people's mind to see what they could avoid ingesting if they will just take five seconds to flip over the package.

I am not advocating, or even talking about, *sugar-free* products. These are still under serious debate regarding artificial sweeteners, so I wouldn't default to buying them. Just stick with low-sugar options.

CONCLUSION

YOU DO YOU.

Today, that phrase means that you do whatever *you* want. But for the purposes of this book, I want you to *do whatever is best for you.* That's really the way to sum up this entire book.

You benefit or *you* suffer from the choices *you* make. No matter if cancer comes flying in from left field or heart disease runs in your family, you have health choices that will absolutely reduce your chances of *additional* pain and suffering. You are the greatest protector of your life and your family. You are the one who determines your future.

> *You* are the one ordering at the restaurant and buying groceries.
>
> *You* are the one using the gym membership, *or not.*
>
> *You* are the one putting on the sunscreen, *or not.*
>
> *You* are the one putting on your seatbelt, your helmet or your condom, *or not.*
>
> *You* are the one that will get melanoma or heart disease or diabetes, *or not.*
>
> *You* will be the one with an unwanted pregnancy, *or not.*
>
> *You* will be the one with a nasty airborne infection, *or not.*
>
> *You* will be the one *dying* from the flu, *or not.*

It's not much different than when you were in school and a teacher caught you cheating. *You were the one* who went to the principal's office. If you ignore the speed limit, *you* get the ticket. But somehow, we think we are going to avoid the penalty of dumb decisions when it comes to unhealthy lifestyle choices.

A friend recently complained that he couldn't figure out if salt was good or bad, whether eggs were good or bad, whether caffeine was good or bad, or which fats were good or bad, so he just declared that none of it really mattered and he ordered the cheesesteak and a beer.

You can absolutely take that approach, *but you are the one that you are affecting.* You are the one that will order the CPAP machine or the oxygen tank or the wheelchair.

There really are good fats and bad fats and they can be confusing, no doubt. But at the end of the day, if you throw in the towel, it's *your body* that will suffer. It's your life that will suck. Sure, your kids and your family and your friends will also suffer the impact of your bad decisions. But you, above all, are the one that will pay the big, nasty, embarrassing, painful price. You are the one to get the pill pack and the needles and the brace and the dentures and the dialysis appointments because you were too cool to wear a seatbelt, stop smoking, apply sunscreen or cut back on the donuts. It's the epitome of insanity to willfully *harm yourself,* but that is what most of us do every single day.

Similarly, you are the one who wins when you can run with your kids or hike or bike. You are the one who wins when you can travel the world instead of traversing the hospital. You win when you invest the thousands of dollars you didn't have to spend on medications. You win when you don't miss the recital or the graduation because you are sick or immobile. You win when you walk into a room with your shoulders back and a healthy glow on your face. You are the one who wins when you prioritize your health, in every decision.

Hopefully, you gleaned a few tips from this book about how to brainlessly build protections into the basic activities of your life, from washing your hands to getting your screenings to exercising. Hopefully, you will default to ordering fruits and vegetables, fish or chicken at a restaurant. Hopefully, you will use sunscreen every day, rain or shine, drink gallons of water, get some healthy sex and sleep like a baby. Most of all, I hope you will never suck on anything that is on fire in your mouth, whether it is a cigarette, a cigar, a hookah, a blunt or a vape.

No matter how much you want to beat the system, fight authority, blame the addiction, look cool, or simply put it off until tomorrow, *you are the one* who will suffer if you do not choose health.

Conversely, you are the one who will experience an extraordinary life of vigor and vitality, health and happiness if you do. So please choose health. I'm rooting for you.

Partial List of References

Allianz Global Assistance

American Academy of Dermatology

American Academy of Family Physicians

American Diabetes Association

ArtandHealing.org

BelieveBig.org

CDC.gov

DavidBach.com

Department of Defense

Divorce Financial Analysts

DoIHavePrediabetes.org

Environmental Working Group

GlobalWorkplaceAnalytics.com

Health.com

HealthLine.com

Hormone Health Network

How To Be Well, Dr. Frank Lipman

Integrated Benefits Institute

Journal of Biological Chemistry

Lonlinessproject.org

TruthInitiative.org

LiveScience.com

Mayo Clinic

NASA, earth data

National Center for Biotechnology Information

PsychologicalScience.org

PsychologyToday.com

Skin Cancer Foundation

Stroke Awareness Foundation

Substance Abuse and Mental Health Services Administration

SugarFixChallenge.org

The Five Love Languages, Gary Chapman

Unlonely Project

WebMD.com

World Health Organization

YouTube.com (23 ½ Hours)

CPSIA information can be obtained
at www.ICGtesting.com
Printed in the USA
LVHW030408210520
656127LV00002B/4/J

9 781646 630240